From Sertão to Surgery

An Orthopaedic Journey

Mark L. Smyth

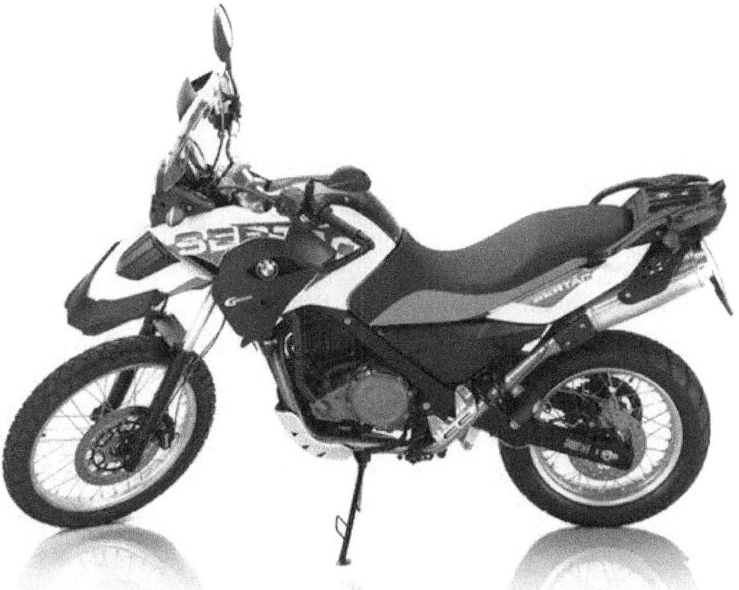

Published in 2015 by:

Mark L. Smyth
Tokyo
Japan
mark@mybritishgarden.com

Printed by CreateSpace, An Amazon.com Company
Available from Amazon and Barnes & Noble Online Stores

Designed and formatted by Mark L. Smyth, Tokyo
Cover design by Mark L. Smyth, Tokyo, using iStudio®

ISBN-13: 978-1502464460

A catalogue record for this book is available from the British Library

In Memory of my Father
Robert Rodger McGregor Smyth
R.I.P.

CONTENTS

Author's Note

Having landed as a patient in a Japanese hospital for three long months would have been difficult enough for any individual but it presented me with greater challenges. As a Westerner, having been a resident in Tokyo for almost twenty years and currently employed as a Senior Consultant within a long-established company, my work mostly involves the training and development of high level executives within large corporate organisations in Tokyo. I had always considered myself fluent in conversational Japanese language skills but all of this is far removed from the world of medicine and I was soon to realise that this Gaijin's (foreigner) comprehension of medical terminology was extremely limited. If I was ever to play a crucial part in my own recovery I had to be clear about the extent of my injuries. I needed to know the nature of my surgeon's proposed treatment and rehabilitation plan. Following my initial trauma and major surgery I not only felt out of action physically but very much out of control mentally. I needed to know what was happening to me and this motivated me, once levitated to a sitting position, to grab my MacBook Air and so began my intense research into the world of medicine throughout my three-month stay in a hospital in Musashikosugi, Kanagawa Prefecture.

Despite my injuries, consequent surgery and post-surgery complications, I threw myself wholeheartedly into my own case study. The very willing and informative hospital Consultants and their teams were happy to discuss the nature of my injuries in detail with me, examining diagrams, and explaining as simply as possible how they intended to repair the extensive damage to my lower leg. During this time I took photos of my X-ray results, my raw injuries, and gathered copious notes in the course of my educational journey. In so doing I felt very much a part of my own healing. Understanding and researching complicated orthopaedic matters was not going to be easy but it kept me motivated and I felt very positive that all of this was a means to success in terms of my recovery and rehabilitation. It was a complicated learning curve for me, a major challenge and with faith in the abilities and skills of the excellent medical staff I proceeded on the journey of a lifetime.

Three months later, on discharge from Kanto Rosai Hospital in Kanagawa, not far from my home in Den-en-Chofu, southern Tokyo, I collated my notes and continued my research into an area which is often a mystery and a wonder to the lay person but holds a particular fascination to me - the world of medicine and surgery.

My personal need had created a burning desire to dig deep into the mass of research information available and to provide a closer look at the medicines prescribed to me, as well as observing at close hand the clinical practices to which I had been subjected during my hospital stay. I felt compelled to share my story with others as I suspect many of us are not entirely *au faire* with the mechanisms of our own bodies and therefore tend to rely on and accept the diagnosis we receive from our doctors; rarely, if ever, questioning the medication prescribed. When something goes wrong with our bodies, be it trauma, pathological disorder, viral infection or some other ailment which befalls us, we feel vulnerable and totally reliant on the medical profession in whose care we are placed.

As a European having resided in Tokyo for a considerable number of years, and having a Japanese wife, I was fairly fluent in the Japanese language but this situation presented great concern when I realized the complexities of medical terminology used within the hospital environment; difficult enough to understand in one's own native language. I wanted to feel in control of my situation and to establish precisely what was happening to me and what was being done to resolve the issues which were unfolding on a daily basis. I immediately put my research skills into practice, armed with technology, and initiated discussions, taking photos and notes with the co-operation (and a degree of fascination) of my doctors who were extremely supportive in my quest.

The Japanese culture appears very conservative and its people seem reluctant to "question authority" as is indeed still the case with many elderly people in the Western world. It follows that the medical staff have limited experience in dealing with patients who wish more in-depth feedback in order to gain a clearer picture of their medical situation. The other communication drawback which presents itself in a patient/doctor situation is the time factor. Many people feel they may be intruding on the doctor's valuable time, while doctors often are, or appear to be, in great demand elsewhere. If this situation was resolved, and time was sufficient to encourage communications, both patient and doctor may well benefit overall in coming to an earlier diagnosis.

I have been as accurate as I can be with regard to surgical procedures which I experienced; fortunate to be able to question the many supportive doctors involved with my case regarding the pre-, per- and post-surgery procedures and the use of equipment and drugs. Other information, e.g., operation timings, were taken directly from hospital logs. Information and data collected by me, re drugs administered orally, intravenously or through inhalation, were confirmed by my doctors and the hospital pharmacists while details on nursing procedures and tasks were confirmed by the nurses who took great care of me during my stay in hospital. With regard to my surgery, I have endeavoured to explain the procedures I experienced in as much detail as I dare, having extracted the "meat of the procedures" from my surgeons as well as from my research findings. Within the context of my book, I have used many medical terms and procedures which are technically descriptive and which may be unfamiliar to the general public. However, I have endeavoured to provide an explanation of the terminology in simplistic form.

Finally, I expect my book will attract various groups of readers; those who know me personally and are, likewise particularly interested in medicine and surgical procedures; medical students seeking specialisms in the fields of orthopaedic surgery and rehabilitation and enthusiastic motorcyclists who understand my dream and who may well have had similar experiences followed by long periods in hospital.

Chapter One
Jiko

I don't recall exactly how I first found myself scrolling the pages on the BMW Motorrad website but however I had arrived, I never looked back. From the moment I began scrolling through the initial pages of information, I was hooked. The opportunity to actually own a BMW motorcycle was an extremely exciting prospect and the more I thought about it, the greater my desire to own one. Perhaps this was indeed what people refer to as a mid life crisis, but I knew in my heart I wanted to relive my younger years. After having spent time perusing their website several times over the course of a week, I decided on the particular model of motorcycle I was going to order. In my younger years, I may well have considered a used motorcycle but now, some twenty-eight years later, I wouldn't settle for anything less than brand new.

The motorcycle I wanted and wanted so badly was the exclusive white BMW g650 GS Sertão, an extremely versatile Enduro motorcycle that would be as happy off-road in the forest tracks below Mount Fuji as it would be on the asphalt roads of Tokyo. I had in actual fact previously considered several other bikes and the hottest contender in that line-up was the four-stroke Kawasaki Ninja 650, all in black, a beautiful bike too in its own class, but the Ninja was just a road bike and many people owned a Kawasaki Ninja. Few people rode BWW Enduro bikes and no biker I ever saw riding on the roads, or even heard of on the bike forums in Japan, talked about owning a g650 GS Sertão. I would be the very proud owner of a very unique bike and for that reason it was a terribly exciting prospect indeed. I spent many hours reading through owner reviews on the Sertão, watching a variety of videos on YouTube and I even went so far as to download a copy of the owner's manual, reading through every single page. There was little doubt in my mind that I had become fairly obsessive about the prospect of owning my own BMW g650 GS Sertão and it may come as no surprise that I was determined to make it happen. I had even considered the possibility of importing directly from the U.K. or U.S., if it came to that. I was in my forties now and this opportunity felt like it might have been my last chance for motorcycle adventure.

Looking back on the calendar, it would have been around the second week in February 2014 that I decided to locate the nearest BMW Motorrad showroom and take a closer look at the actual bike. Fortunately, I discovered from their website that there was a showroom not far from Tokyo Haneda International Airport, on Kanpachi Road, about a twenty minute drive from home and so one sunny afternoon, I took a drive out there after exchanging a few emails with Mr. Takeo Satoh, the company Chief Executive Officer (CEO). To some, that may sound a little odd, being in direct contact with a CEO over a single sales enquiry but this is Japan! Aside from doing things differently to that which many of us may be used to in our home countries, as a foreigner and a native English speaker I often get to deal with the person who can speak my language, which means I usually find myself dealing with the management directly. I hadn't told Mr. Satoh in our email exchange that I was particularly interested in the g650 GS Sertão, I enquired if he had any Enduro bikes in stock and he kindly welcomed me to his showroom. As a courtesy, I informed him that I planned on visiting the showroom some three days later, to ascertain if he would be available.

When that day arrived, there was not a single cloud and the sun was sitting high up in the clear blue sky. Perfect weather for my journey. As I left the house, securely locking the door behind me, I made my way down the grey tiled concrete steps adjacent to the sandstone wall of the garden next door. As a keen gardener with little space to indulge my hobby, I had softened in appearance the blandness of the gable-end wall with climbing ivy and a pretty young sprouting buddleia which was now beginning to blossom. Stepping out of the shadow of the sandstone wall, past the array of terra cotta pots of pink, blue and yellow geraniums, I felt the sudden warmth of the sun on my face. The street was almost empty except for two fashionably dressed Japanese women on the other side, holding delicately onto their black frilly parasols to shade them from the direct sun.

I turned towards the garage and reaching into the right hand pocket of my black leather jacket, I pulled out the car key fob and clicking the button on it, unlocked the central locking system in my white Mercedes which responded with a familiar clunk. The car was facing nose first into the cool shadow of the garage, where I edged my way down the right hand side and opened the driver's door. The smell of lavender from the car air freshener greeted me pleasantly. After programming the car navigation system, I pulled the seatbelt over my shoulder, switched on the hazard warning lights, which is customary in Japan, clicked the automatic gearbox shift down into reverse and slowly backed out of the cool shade of the garage, across the red bricked pavement and onto the road. From the beech trees lining the park I could hear the constant buzzing of cicadas. Then, clicking the gearbox into drive I followed the winding slope down towards the railway crossing some 200 metres at the bottom of the street.

I stopped at the thick white line in front of the crossing and made a positive visual scan left and right along the empty train line before moving swiftly over the two sets of lines. I was particularly careful with this manoeuvre having previously been fined by a police officer positioned on the opposite side of the crossing, as if waiting like a lion ready to pounce on all the prey who failed to stop and carry out this action.

When I reached the other side of the crossing, I could see several more people walking between Tamagawa Station, around a hundred metres to my right and the bus terminal just to my left, in front of Tamagawa Swimming Pool. There was also a young female kindergarten teacher wearing the traditional yellow full length apron, pushing a four-wheeled cart, caged on all four sides, along the footpath with half a dozen kindergarten children in it, a reminder of one of the safe practices carried out in this country.

Directly ahead of me, across the Tamagawa River, I could clearly see in the near distance, the high rise apartments of the vastly expanding town of

Musashikosugi. When the traffic lights changed to green, I turned left and joined the main road alongside the Tamagawa River, its rippling waters flowing gently under the distinctive blue painted iron engineering of Marukobashi Bridge immediately to my right.

The Tamagawa is a long river, some one hundred and thirty eight kilometres in length and flows all the way from its source at Mount Kasadori in Yamanashi Prefecture in the Chubu region west of the capital, through the dam in Okutama National Park and forming the divide between Tokyo and Kanagawa, it continues until it reaches Tokyo Bay by the side of Haneda International Airport. On both sides of the river, sports teams can be seen on a regular basis practicing a range of sports including rugby, football and baseball. Golf driving ranges, playgrounds and parking facilities are available where the river passes through the city. Other popular sports and activities include kayaking, white water rafting and hydro-speeding on the river which are run by many companies from early Spring until late Autumn, all activities, competitions and events being easily accessible from Tokyo city. Many people escaping the bustle of city life and looking for a more tranquil relaxing break will take advantage of the easy-to-ride cycle paths, taking a leisurely cycle ride down meandering paths while enjoying the scenery, taking in the life of this magnificent river and enjoying respite from the crowds.

I observed on my route, a police box, manned by two Metropolitan police officers in their standard uniform of blue button-down shirt, trousers and stab vest, who appeared to be asking questions of a casually dressed young Japanese male who was holding on to a bicycle. I wondered if he had been suspected of stealing the bicycle as his body language suggested to me he was feeling rather uncomfortable. Further along the road I could see two men and a woman who appeared to be in their early thirties, jogging together. They were dressed in Nike and Mizuno tops and running tights, with water belts around their waists. Many people use this road alongside the Tamagawa River as it provides a pleasant environment for fitness exercise.

Driving on past telegraph poles holding up more than a dozen cables running alongside the road, I couldn't help but wonder why Tokyo did not hide all these electrical cables underground as is practice in the U.K. The lines themselves run close in front of a mishmash of buildings of varying heights, colours and styles, on either side of these busy roads. I checked the car mirrors again and moved into the right hand lane, indicating my intention to turn right under the underpass, in order to join the main road above. As the overhead traffic lights showed a green arrow pointing right, I was able to continue the manoeuvre and follow on the slip road that ran alongside Kanpachi Road above. On either side, there were pedestrians and people on shopping bikes, referred to as '*Mama Charis*', waiting to cross one of four zebra crossings. This is a junction system unseen in the U.K. which consists of a series of straight, continuous and curved broken lines serving as lane guides for the two lanes of traffic. If the lights are on green, you are allowed to pull forward, following the right curve which brings you up to a point where you can see oncoming traffic. From here you can judge if it is safe to continue your turn to join the slip road on the right. If the lights display a green arrow, then you are safe to proceed as the traffic on the opposite side would be stopped to give way.

Soon, I joined the gently upward sloping slip road that ran alongside Kanpachi Road above. On the left hand side, the pavement was much wider, and there were pedestrians and people on shopping bikes going about their business. I carefully joined the faster flowing traffic on this busy three-lane road.

Kanpachi Road is a busy road and this particular stretch was running towards Haneda International Airport. I had now several cars passing me on the outside lane and a large goods vehicle directly behind me. In front of me was a small white van with a yellow number plate. In Japan, most vehicles have white number plates, front and rear. However, there are a significant number of vehicles with yellow number plates. These vehicles are in the K-Class, referred to as *Kei Cars* (meaning "light automobile") and have engines smaller than 1000cc. Kei cars are quite popular with small businesses and, aside from being easier to drive around the narrow backstreets of the Tokyo suburbs, are a lot easier to park as they are quite small.

There was also a multitude of cables running alongside this road and although the road itself was a little wider than the previous roads, there was still a continuing mishmash of different buildings. However, this time there was a greater number of medium sized apartment blocks dotted between the variety of car showrooms, ramen restaurants, pizza parlours and the odd golf equipment shop. Under the electric cables were equally spaced and well-cropped ginko trees, their foul smelling nuts strewn by the roadside and crushed by passing tyres, leaving a sticky mess across the road.

As I continued for another twenty minutes along Kanpachi Road, I reached the crossing by the side of Otorii Station, the main railway station that serves this area, its lines rising above the surrounding chaos of buildings, people, parked bicycles and the busy traffic below. My destination was just up ahead and as I neared the familiar BMW logo, I slowed down and turned left, negotiating my way over the pavement, rolling into one of two parking slots at the side of the building. I had finally arrived at BMW Motorrad Haneda.

The showroom itself was fairly large, with a series of tall glass panes and an ample area at the front where several motorcycles were parked. BMW Motorrad Haneda occupied the whole of the ground space underneath a large apartment block. As I walked into the showroom I felt a sense of excitement wash over me. It reminded me of a moment, many years ago when I visited a Yamaha showroom in northern Scotland to purchase my first motorcycle; a black, water-cooled Yamaha DT125LC trail bike. The similarity quickly faded though as I turned to experience the richness and ambience of what lay before me. Unlike the smaller Yamaha motorcycles I had gone to see all those years ago, here I found myself surrounded by more than twenty brand new large engine BMW bikes on show. For a brief moment, time appeared to slow down. In my awe, I wanted to take time to wander through the variety of machines around me, but just then, Mr. Satoh emerged from his office door at the back of the reception area and with a welcoming smile upon his face, immediately extended a hand to greet me. Much to my delight, this gentleman proved capable of communicating reasonably well in English and thanked me for 'troubling myself' to visit his showroom.

Mr. Satoh was approximately 180cm tall, around his mid-sixties and as I soon discovered, loved riding BMWs. After we exchanged some small talk, he introduced me to a white BMW g650 GS which was sitting on a vertical showroom stand in front of a rack displaying BMW equipment catalogues. This was the base model for the Sertão, but it wasn't the actual g650 GS Sertão, the bike modeled on the former BMW Dakar. There were undoubtedly a lot of similarities between these two models, but the immediate impression one would get looking at both models side by side is that the g650 GS, with it's slick tyres and aluminium wheels was that this bike was more of a road bike, whereas the g650 GS Sertão with it's adventurous decals and spoked wheels was built for the trails. Nevertheless, I took a good look at the bike and after one of his sales advisors kindly rolled the bike clear of the others on either side, I was able to mount the bike and see how it felt for size. I am 186cm tall, with reasonably long legs and this was a fairly high bike, but it fitted me well. Gripping the handlebars and with my feet on the pegs, I felt very comfortable and confident I could handle its size.

My treatment in the showroom was a prime example of the quality shopping experience in Japan. As a customer, you are always treated with respect and ultimate attention. Japan should be proud of its high quality customer service. Whenever you walk into a shop in Japan, you are greeted and made to feel very welcome. The shop assistant or owner is always happy to attend to your needs and listen carefully to you, without troubling you and making you feel pressurised. Even if you decide not to purchase anything, you will be thanked for visiting as you leave.

Here, inside the showroom of BMW Motorrad Haneda I was being treated to an experience which made me feel confident, important and totally relaxed. After looking at several models, Mr. Satoh introduced me to the new BMW 4-stroke twin-cylinder engine F700 GS so I could draw a comparison with the single cylinder g650 GS. The F700 GS was also a nice bike and it had some features, like digital engine management and the larger capacity fuel tank that I liked, but I told Mr. Satoh what I was particularly interested in viewing was the BMW g650 GS Sertão. I was rather disappointed to hear that he didn't have one in the showroom, but given my desire to purchase this particular bike, he asked his Sales Manager, Mr. Masahiro Nozaka to check the Japan BMW Motorrad database right away. While I waited, Mr. Satoh's secretary brought me a cup of freshly brewed coffee in a delicate white porcelain cup and saucer, together with a little jug of fresh single cream and a small sugar bowl containing several lumps of brown cane sugar.

We chatted for a little while, during which time I informed Mr. Satoh that I was still doing the 'Ogata' or 'Large Motorcycle' course at driving school and as yet had not been awarded the relevant motorcycle licence. I added that my test would be coming up two weeks later and my instructors (all Examiners) were confident I would pass. I had been told that the test was really a confirmation of the high level of riding skills I had already achieved and provided I didn't make any major mistakes during the actual test itself I would be awarded this certificate. For those readers outside Japan, this reassurance may sound at the very least, unusual, however, it is a custom in Japan for such retailers to expect this provisional notice so that they can market their products, especially to potential motorcycle licence holders. With a reassuring smile across his face, Mr. Satoh told me that it would not be a problem as the actual sale could be arranged a little later when I received my licence. Furthermore, he informed me that BMW Motorrad Japan was running a campaign that offered students of the Ogata course a very attractive discount if they initiated the purchase of a new bike. Any sale of course is subject to receipt of the official Ogata licence.

We had been chatting for around twenty minutes or so when Mr. Nozaka finally stood up from the computer screen behind the sales desk and was pleased to inform me that, according to the central database, there were only two new models of the Sertão available in the whole of Japan. I wanted one of them and so Mr. Nozaka placed a reservation on one of the bikes which was in a showroom in Hokkaido, the northernmost island in Japan. I had 30 days on this reservation by which time I would be able to confirm award of my certificate/licence. I duly signed the provisional paperwork for the reservation and verbally agreed to transfer a 10% deposit within the next few days, which would be refundable in the event I had not gained my licence. I felt very excited about my potential purchase. The Sertão was an expensive purchase but I was confident I would have no regrets. Mr. Satoh was particularly happy to do business with me after discovering we were in fact neighbours.

On the morning of the day I headed out to pick up my new Sertão, I was elated. I had travelled to the BMW showroom by car on the first occasion as it was simply more convenient. However, obviously given the fact that I'd have to ride back home, I needed to take the train this time.

Prior to leaving the house I double checked that I had my black Nitro helmet with flip-up visor, black Viper waterproof textile fabric motorcycle trousers and my Oakley kevlar-backed motorcycle gloves, all carefully packed into my black Mountain Hardware backpack. I was already wearing my black leather motorcycle jacket and leather boots. I turned the key and locked the door, once again moving down and out of the shadow of sandstone and ivy to the sunshine glaring through the gaps in the tree branches above me as I made my way down the hill towards the station. There were a few more people on the street this particular afternoon; a woman walking two little dogs the size of two large rats and two schoolgirls in navy blue uniform riding bicycles. I noticed an old man walking along the edge of the road smoking a cigarette, the cancerous smoke bellowing from his lungs, which I duly avoided by crossing the street. As I approached the railway crossing at the bottom of the road, I turned immediately right, following the path which ran alongside the Tamagawa railway line, passing several more people along the way.

To the left of the path were around a hundred or so bicycles neatly parked between the painted white lines that divided the parking spaces, patrolled by the local warden. As this was also a bicycle-parking area, the local Council had thought it a good idea to install a series of staggered white painted metal barriers to stop cyclists actually riding along the path, but it had almost the reverse effect. Cyclists still rode, but slower, and pedestrians became even more inconvenienced as they often had to stop to give way to bicycles or other pedestrians.

As I neared the station, I could hear the trains overhead as they approached and left the station, their steel wheels screeching along the iron railway lines. With my *'Passmo'* contact-less rail card, I passed through the ticket barrier and made my way down towards the Tamagawa Line, a line that starts at Tamagawa Station and terminates at Kamata, the ten-minute ride making it one of Tokyo's shortest rail journeys.

The train was fairly packed as usual so when I reached Kamata and the train doors were simultaneously opened by the driver, I alighted and, together with the crowd I was caught up in, headed towards the row of ticket barriers which we all had to pass through. On the other side of the ticket barriers and amidst the confusion of people, there were a number of small shops and the entrance to Tokyu Department Store that sat to the side and above the station. As I made my way along the side of the department store, the conglomeration of aromas drifted pleasantly up my nostrils. I passed a shop selling freshly cooked pancakes, another selling Japanese green tea, a shop selling hot sugared bagels and another selling freshly baked bread. There was a coffee shop which released the welcoming aroma of constant coffee bean brewing and another shop selling hot steamed Chinese gyoza, a spicy mix of ground meat and vegetables, wrapped in a thin dough. I was beginning to feel hungry as I walked past all these tempting smells. I made my way down the escalator and through the large automated glass doors which slid open as I approached them and on the next step of my journey I was able to navigate the streets of Kamata between Kamata Station and Keikyukamata Station, a flat walk of around fifteen minutes.

The streets around the southern side of Kamata Station were less narrow and congested with shoppers than those of the northern side but nevertheless, there were plenty of people walking around and the cars on the road added to the quaintness of this bustling old shopping town. Navigating along the street, relying on the accuracy of the Google Maps app on my iPhone, I felt confident in reaching my destination. As I wound through the variety of small, often narrow streets, I came across the tall car parking towers so unique to Japan, the noisy pachinko parlours, ramen and sushi restaurants, a mini supermarket and an array of small bars scheduled to open only in the evenings.

Suddenly, I heard the familiar sound of a train close by which was crossing high up from the road on which I was traveling. This elevated train line had been the result of a long-awaited railway project designed to reduce the traffic congestion below caused by several light-controlled railway crossings along the line. I could see Keikyukamata Station perched high above on this line, the sides of which were painted in a creamy yellow colour and the entrance at the base, resembling the entrance to a huge spaceship hovering above with it's ramp lowered. This was a new, modern, spacious station and I followed the incredibly long escalator to the top where I proceeded through the ticket barriers and made my way to Platform Two.

There were few people waiting for the train but when it arrived, the whole train emptied itself of passengers, temporarily disturbing the relative calm of the station. In this orderly country, there are always painted lines to be found marked on the platform. These lines indicate where the doors will open so that passengers waiting for a train know exactly where to stand. If, on such a rare occasion, the train does not align with these markings, particularly if the platform has additional safety doors, the passengers need not move as the train driver will either pull the train forward a little or reverse until the doors are aligned with these markings, at the same time apologising to the passengers on board for missing the alignment on the first attempt. Most of the time though drivers are skilled enough to stop the train precisely at the same point each time.

With the exception of the Shinkansen and Narita Express trains, the seats on the majority of trains in Tokyo are long fabric padded benches facing each other, intended to both maximise the number of passengers by allowing many people to stand while gripping the handrails above and to allow passengers to move through the train more easily.

It took only a few minutes to reach Otorii Station but my final destination was a good ten minutes walk from there. The road was as busy as it always is and so too was the flow of pedestrians and people riding bicycles on the pavement. It is actually against the law to ride a bicycle on a pedestrian walkway but the police generally do not bother to enforce this law on cyclists in Japan.

Finally I reached my destination, arriving at the BMW Motorrad showroom, where I was warmly greeted by Mr. Satoh who congratulated me on gaining my Ogata licence. I then signed the relevant paperwork and insurance policy for my new Sertão. On completion of the administration, Mr. Satoh had one of his sales advisors, Mr. Toshiaki Nakada wheel my new bike out of the showroom and park it up at the side of the main road. I was naturally anxious about riding my new powerful purchase as this would be my first time with my new bike on a public road and it wasn't by any means a quiet one. With a total length of 44.2 km (27.5 miles), Kanpachi Dori (literal translation 'Ring Road no.8') is a metropolitan road connecting Tokyo Haneda International Airport in Ota Ward and Iwabuchi-cho, in Kita Ward, making it one of the busiest roads in suburban Tokyo.

Nevertheless, after donning my motorcycle trousers, my helmet and gloves, I fastened my backpack to my back and gripping some courage, prepared to mount my new motorbike. Even though I have long legs, the Sertão is a tall bike and as I took hold of the handlebars and swung my right leg over the bike seat, the heel of my boot caught the rear access panel and ripped off a small design strip. Mr. Satoh insisted that his staff would fix it and asked me to ride the bike around the back of the building where the workshop was located. I followed his instructions and parked up in front of the workshop entrance. Mr. Satoh had in the meantime walked through the back of the showroom to meet me and had one of his staff epoxy it back in position.

When I finally rode off, I decided to ride for a while around the back streets to get used to the bike, particularly clutch bite and throttle control, for these are undoubtedly the most essential controls to master on any manual bike. I was exceptionally impressed with the braking system. All the time spent on the various bikes I had been riding, I needed to master the pressure and graduation of braking, particularly during emergency braking practice, in order to avoid skidding and losing control of the bike, but now I had ABS literally at my fingertips. I loved it. It was now practically impossible to skid and what's more, the ABS system on the Sertão is switchable, meaning that you can leave it on while riding on-road but switch it off when heading off-road. In addition to the ABS, there was a three position switch to activate the heated handlebar grips, a fabulous extra in cold weather.

I initially rode around for two hours or so, during which time I passed small parks where mothers were playing with their children on the swings and a few pedestrians as they walked by on the street. I rode past a multitude of small houses, each one different from the other in both colour and architecture. I saw school students riding bicycles and I passed small businesses, some selling bread, others selling vegetables, sometimes extending their goods out into the street. There were convenience stores along the way and an astounding number of vending machines selling hot and cold drinks. I stopped often at the small crossroads that dotted the one-way streets adorning suburban Tokyo. Sitting high on my new "horse", I could hear the imaginary voices of the pedestrians I passed, call out *"Look! a BMW g650 GS Sertão!"* and *"Wow! Cool bike!"* More than one year had passed since I initiated pursuit of my dream and here it was, the very moment had at long last, been realised. All the pieces of the jigsaw were finally coming together to complete the whole picture.

However, at this stage my dream was *not entirely* complete as I had originally attached a condition. I would only purchase the bike after having purchased all the motorcycle gear first, and not just any gear, I wanted the best. I wanted BMW Motorrad original motorcycle clothing, designed for BMW Enduro riding. I had browsed the Motorrad website and had a copy of the clothing catalogue. I knew exactly what clothing I wanted. I planned to order the GS range of Enduro clothing, jacket, trousers, helmet, gloves and GS Enduro boots that would totally protect the bottom half of my legs. However, the drawback here was that I am a 186cm tall Westerner in Japan and as such it is difficult to find any clothing in my size, as Japanese sizes are somewhat smaller. That applies to both casual and business. I have little choice but to purchase practically all my clothing from my home country, Scotland, whenever I visit there. The BMW clothing I wanted to buy was also not available in my size in

Japan so consequently the shop would arrange to have it imported directly from BMW in Germany and that would take time. So in the meantime, I would ride around with alternative, but suitable clothing, something I would later regret.

Waiting until I could have all the BMW clothing first before ordering the bike went out the window when I discovered the rarity of the Sertão in Japan, even more so now that BMW Motorrad Japan have apparently stopped importing single cylinder bikes. The bike came first and it was a matter of placing a special order for the clothing and wait for it to arrive.

There was, however, one last, rather important issue related to the bike and that was where to park this big machine. As there were no parking spots nearby in my neighbourhood, the parking spot I had no choice but to use, was actually my home theatre. That must sound really strange but to throw some perspective on the situation, I considered at first parking the bike in the garage, underneath the house, but the car took all the space up, so parking there was out of the question. Nor was it possible or practical to park at the rear of the car. A few years previously, I had built a sound-proof room out of reinforced concrete block and wood, at the back of the garage to use as a home theatre. This room extended the three metre width of the garage and was two and a half metres deep. I'd raised the floor ten centimetres off the concrete floor of the garage so that I could install an insulation course under the white oak flooring. The other reason for raising the floor was that as the flooring level extended out of the room door and about one metre back into the garage, it would also serve as a guide and stop for the front tyres of the car when I was parking. This meant I could park the nose of the car just centimetres from the wall of my room, maximising the limited space I had. This, therefore, was the only place I could park the bike.

I had meticulously measured the available space in the room and confirmed and re-confirmed the dimensions of the bike before purchase. I was confident the bike would fit inside the room, but what I could not confirm until I had actually bought the bike was whether or not it would fit through the slightly larger than normal sized doorframe into the room. The doorframe width is 74cm. The handlebars, and thereby the widest point on the bike, were 92cm. I knew at the back of my mind I could make it fit somehow. Ninety Two centimetres was the width the handlebars took up when the front wheel was pointing forward, but when the wheel was on full lock either way, the width they took up was reduced to 82cm. So there was a definite art to getting the bike into the room, without damaging the doorframe, door or walls inside, or the bike itself for that matter.

In order to get it into the room and parked at almost ninety degrees from the position it had entered, I had to set a small ramp onto the ten centimetre high floor, thereby bridging the height difference and then manoeuvre the left hand grip past the door frame first, gradually lean the bike to the left until the right hand grip could clear the opposite side of the door frame and push what felt like a stubborn cow halfway into the room, at the same time continuing a right hand turn until it reached the wood panelling on the end wall. Then, I needed to grip the rear end of the bike and bump it up and down to swing the back end around, as it was practically impossible to lift the almost two hundred kilograms of machine, until I could change the angle so that the rear end cleared the path of the door, allowing it to be closed. In this position, I had tried to use the side stand but that made the bike lean over about forty degrees which made it impossible to park without it leaning against my digital fireplace. The solution was to build a temporary wooden box for the engine to rest up against, allowing the bike to be parked upright. It sounds like an awful lot of trouble just to park a bike and it was at first but I did it so many times that it eventually didn't take long to accomplish the task.

In the following weeks I continued to enjoy riding the bike around town. I rode as far uptown as Nihonbashi, around Tokyo Station, Ikebukuro and Shibuya and soon I clocked up one thousand kilometers, at which point my Sertão enjoyed her first service. During the second thousand kilometers, I often rode along the scenic road that ran atop the embankment of the Tamagawa River up to Futakotamagawa in the west and then back eastwards on the other side of the river, across into Kawasaki, before heading back home across the familiar blue structure of Marukobashi bridge. These were not terribly long journeys as such and I really wanted to travel further afield, somewhere like the rolling hills of Hokkaido Island in northern Japan, but the hour or hour and a half journeys taught me something valuable. They taught me how desperately I needed a new seat.

There are three seat heights available for the Sertão and perhaps not surprisingly, I discovered that for the Japan market, BMW bikes were fitted with the smallest height seats. No wonder my rear end was so uncomfortable. It would have been total agony to attempt a journey more than two or three hours. I needed the tallest seat, known as the Sertão Dakar seat, named after the Sertão's predecessor, the BMW Dakar, but the seat would come after the safety clothing.

The month of May seemed to pass by quickly and the arrival of June now marked the beginning of the warm, humid season and the approach to the pre-summer *'tsuyu'*, or rainy season, which can bring torrential rain to Japan. It was warm and humid and I was starting to sweat under my motorcycle clothing. People would ask me why I would wear such *'winter-looking'* clothing in such warm weather but my question in Tokyo, following observations, was why in Summer would anyone with any sense be riding a scooter or motorcycle with a helmet that barely covered the skull, a T-shirt, no gloves and flip flops, and sometimes a similarly dressed "chick" on the back? I'd rather sweat than end up in hospital!

Chapter Two
Kyūkyūsha

On the morning of Thursday, 5th June, 2014, I did have the grave misfortune to end up in hospital. I had always demonstrated safe riding skills ever since being released onto the public road system. My g650 GS Sertão was a reasonably tall bike and as a result I found myself sat upright in a position high enough to see over the top of much of the traffic. I made a point of keeping safe distance between the traffic, front and rear, so that if I did need to use the ABS in an emergency, I would be able to stop clear of the vehicle in front and the distance I maintained with the vehicle behind me would ensure that I could manoeuvre to the side, should the vehicle behind need to brake hard. I never failed to check the mirrors and was aware of the traffic situation around me at all times. I never meandered in and out of the traffic as many scooter and motorcycle riders do in Tokyo and if I did need to pass alongside any vehicle, for example at traffic lights, I always knew when I was in the drivers' blind spot, especially large trucks. I would obey the speed limits, pay special attention at railway crossings and every time I planned to make a turn or avoid a hazard, I would do a mirror check to indicate to drivers behind that I was likely to make a move, and then indicate a few seconds before, followed by a shoulder check, or "lifesaver" as it's sometimes called, before actually executing the manoeuvre. I never intentionally ventured out into the rain but if it happened to rain while I was riding, I would reduce my speed accordingly, to match the road conditions. During my large motorcycle training course at KDS, one of my instructors, Mr. Noboru Kato, gave me plenty of good advice, but one particular piece of advice he gave me stuck with me. He told me how riders of large motorcycles, and therefore holders of the ogata licence, should see themselves. He said that holding an ogata licence was a privilege and being the highest category of licence, those riders should be proud to demonstrate to all lesser qualified riders, sensible riding. However, it was none of that sensible, safe riding that put me in hospital. What landed me in the operating theatre was a freak accident and the "freak" in it was about to change the course of my life.

At 09:45 on the morning of that Thursday, a fair, dry day, I reversed the car out of the garage and parked it halfway up onto the red bricked pavement so

I could wheel my bike out of its comfortable parking space and clear of the garage. I parked it up in the usual place, the only place it was stable, on the pavement, slightly up the slope from the entrance to the garage and as close to the three-metre sandstone wall of my next door neighbour as I could, making sure the 21″ spoked front wheel was securely up against the one metre high blue-grey slate stone wall of my water garden, by the side of the garage, so there was no chance it would roll off its side stand. Not only was the pavement on a slope but it was also chamfered in towards the one way road. Not the greatest place to park a two hundred kilogram motorcycle but there was absolutely nowhere else available.

I had already donned my motorcycle trousers, protective leather jacket and boots, so after returning the car to the garage and greeting the apartment manager of the condominium next to my house who was busy sweeping the area clear of fallen leaves, I walked uphill towards my bike. When I reached my bike, I pulled on my leather and kevlar gloves and slipped my helmet over my head, clicking the chinstrap together and flipping up the visor. Maintaining a firm grip on the handlebars and the front brake lever, I mounted the bike. With my left foot firmly on the ground and my right foot balanced on my toes, I pulled slightly backwards to free the front wheel from the wall of my water garden, then pulled in the front brake to stop this big machine from freewheeling down the hill. Before I rolled towards the roadside though, I had to confirm that there were no pedestrians walking down the hill behind me, nor cars coming down the hill, so I stole a glance in the right hand mirror. I couldn't see any cars and there was no one walking down on my side of the footpath. I checked over my shoulder to confirm that situation as I normally would but as I returned my head to the front again, I suddenly lost my balance.

It happened so quickly that I had absolutely no chance to recover the bike from the inevitable. Still in the seat and holding on to the handlebars, I went straight down with the bike and although I got thrown outward a little due to the chamfering of the road, the bike came down hard and fast a split second later right on top of the lower half of my right leg. For what seemed like no more than a mere second or two, I was aglow with complete embarrassment for having lost control of this powerful machine and no less so for having done it right in front of the house. The bike was lying down on the pavement and I was lying on the road.

The feeling of embarrassment vanished just as quickly when I realised that my right foot was at a most unusual angle. I knew then that I had broken my leg. Due to the black Viper motorcycle trousers I was wearing, I was unable to see that the tibia and fibula bones in my right leg had been forced out of my flesh though there was absolutely no doubt I could feel the resulting pain. Suddenly I found myself hurled into a world of shock and excruciating pain. I felt completely helpless as I lay there on the road, calling out "Itaaaiii! Ashi ga itai!", the Japanese version of "It hurts! My leg hurts!" Certain Japanese words are easier to use than English and "itai" was one of those words. I lay there, gritting my teeth in the ridiculous hope that it might create sufficient distraction to absorb some of the pain. It was a natural reaction to such a shocking incident. I simply couldn't believe what had just happened; going from a simple mirror check whilst sat on my bike, to lying on the road below in absolute agony a few seconds later. It still sends a shiver down my spine whenever I recall that moment.

The apartment manager did not actually witness me go down as he had his back to me at the time but he most certainly heard me. It must have been quite a shock for him too. He dropped his brush and rushed up the slope to help me, along with a middle-aged Japanese lady who happened to be passing by at that point. There were very few people walking by at that time as the area is a reasonably quiet residential area and rush-hour had well passed, but another man whom I later learned was the water meter reader for the six-floored apartment block next door, rushed to my aid. What felt like just a few seconds later, another couple of people rushed over to this now desperate scene. In my utterly helpless state, I felt a dire sense of dependency on these people whose day I had interrupted. With my leg obviously broken, I was unable to even sit up but they helped drag me to the side of the road in case any cars were to come down the hill.

Obviously someone had called an ambulance and while waiting for it to arrive, the apartment manager and one of the men tried to lift my bike, and not without great difficulty. There is a particular skill for just one person to lift a large motorcycle and only a motorcyclist would know how to do that without too much of a struggle. Eventually though, they managed to return my bike upright with all the strength they had, but now I was immensely concerned that it would fall over again or just as disastrous, roll off its side stand and roll back onto the road. Amidst the pain and gritting of teeth, I asked them to make sure the ignition key was turned all the way to the left so as to lock the front wheel and to ensure the front tyre was firmly up against the water garden. That was imperative, no matter what.

While the two men struggled to lift my bike, the lady who was crouched down beside me tried to reassure me and even did so in her somewhat limited English. I am truly grateful to the apartment manager and to those strangers who came to my aid that morning and I hope one day to have the opportunity to thank them all.

I heard the unmistakable sound of the ambulance siren a couple of blocks away just five or six minutes later and by the time it arrived, a few more people had gathered on the scene, including a couple of neighbours from the apartment block on the north east side of my house. Although I was the real victim, I couldn't help but feel apologetic for having my neighbours see me in such a shocking situation as I was lifted onto a collapsible trolley by the two attending paramedics and slid into the 4WD 5-door Toyota Himedic ambulance. I gave a thumbs up to Mrs. Ushio, the apartment owner next door to reassure her I was relatively okay, given what had just happened.

As the tailgate of the ambulance was closed, I thought the vehicle would speed off straight away to hospital, but instead it drove just a few metres further down the road and parked halfway up onto the pavement. One of the paramedics took out a flexible metal splint, shaped like a small ladder and placed it alongside the posterior of my entire leg, bending the metal frame so that it followed the least painful position, but every tiny movement just hurt more. It was necessary to attach this splint to my leg somehow, in order to stabilise my injury and this he achieved by tying strips of white cotton cloth around both my leg and the splint. After stabilising my leg, he asked me if I'd like to call my wife, Noriko, and let her know that I'd had an accident and was being taken to hospital. Probably due to the shock of the accident, I couldn't bring myself to speak to her directly, so I dialed her number from my contacts and passed the phone over. When he had finished informing her, the side door slid open and a police officer dressed in navy blue uniform with a flat peaked hat and a pistol in the holster by his waist, entered the vehicle to confirm my name and address as he jotted down some details on the A4 plastic clipboard he was holding. At the time, that seemed ridiculous, given that the accident happened right outside my house. He also wanted me to confirm briefly what had happened. Considering the pain I was in, I was quite frustrated at this delay, but I later learned that the apartment manager had kindly called out the police to help confirm the accident to my insurance company. That was particularly thoughtful of him.

When the ambulance finally drove off, it bumped down off the kerb which just served to intensify my pain, as did every road surface imperfection on the way to the hospital. I couldn't help myself from calling out in pain and gritting my teeth to hold back the tears. It's hard to imagine now that I was in so much pain. That was, doubtless, the worst pain I have ever experienced in my life. In the past few years, I've fractured my big toe with the chrome 'safety' bar on a Honda CBR 400, ripped the entire nail off my first finger with a Bosch PBS-75A belt sander and pulled the raw flesh halfway up my finger with a strip of aluminium railing. However, as shocking as these accidents were, I was able to handle the pain with dignity and even had time to take a few shots with my iPhone for my personal memory album. I assumed the ambulance would be heading for Den-en-chofu Central Hospital, just a few minutes drive away, although if given a choice I'd have opted for the longer journey to Sanno Hospital, a bilingual, modern hospital in Aoyamaitchome in uptown Tokyo that resembles a hotel inside. It was there that Doctor Kurashima, a fluent English speaking otolaryngologist with a good sense of humour, had performed my nasal septoplasty. This is also the hospital I attend for a routine health check on an annual basis where I enjoy chatting to Dr. Monzen, a very knowledgeable doctor, who is fluent in English.

However, after a while, it was apparent that we were heading further away than the local hospital, although, for once in my life, navigation was not top of the agenda and consequently I had no bearing or idea where we were heading. Being reasonably familiar now with the journey, I'd calculate that approximately ten minutes must have passed before we reached the destination hospital. As the ambulance approached the entrance, an automated recorded alert calmly came over the vehicle loudspeaker *"Kyūkyūsha ga migi e magarimasu"* meaning "The ambulance is turning right". As it made its turn into the entrance, the siren was silenced and the ambulance reversed up towards the building. When the frosted glass tailgate swung up, I could see a set of metal double doors wide open and several nurses coming out to wheel me into the Emergency Room beyond. Still in immense pain, I managed to blurt out *"Ohayo Gozaimasu"*, meaning "Good Morning". This was quickly becoming a surreal moment for me. I felt as if I were the main actor in a television hospital drama, only I was not acting. This was a real Emergency Room and I was experiencing real pain. As for which hospital it actually was I still had not the foggiest idea.

The E.R. doctor on duty that day was Doctor Akira Tsuchiya, an Orthopaedic Surgeon in his early thirties. It was obvious he spoke little English, just the odd short sentence and several single words. I'm sure he wasn't ready for someone like me, a foreigner , or "*gaijin*" who had just been rushed into a totally Japanese environment. However, although I was physically in pain, I was comfortable communicating in Japanese: I just wished the pain to subside. Dr. Tsuchiya immediately administered intravenous Fentanyl at a concentration of 2ml. Fentanyl is a narcotic analgesic and works in the brain and nervous system to cause anaesthesia and decrease pain. In the E.R. that day, it was used for both alleviating my pain and for initiating the primary stage of anaesthesia for my surgery. As I lay there, on the trolley, still wearing my boots and motorcycle clothing, I waited with intense impatience for this painkilling drug to take effect while Dr. Tsuchiya closely monitored its efficacy in order to determine whether it was working properly and if I should continue to receive this particular drug.

It must have taken around twenty minutes before the fentanyl registered any noticeable effect, but it never fully suppressed the pain. By the time my wife, Noriko had arrived, the worst of the pain had subsided. Dr. Tsuchiya then informed me that it would take around two hours before I could be operated on.

Such a length of time played on my mind while I lay there waiting. Two hours waiting for a friend in Starbucks is a reasonably long wait but two hours waiting for an emergency operation would prove to be an incredibly torturous experience. I flashed back through my life to the many times in which I had to wait for two hours. I recalled waiting for a bus in the Lake District in England to take me to Newcastle, waiting on a grassy hilltop in sunny Saitama, Japan for the wind to increase enough to raise my canopy at paragliding school; waiting at the incredibly bustling hub of Schiphol International Airport in Amsterdam, for my connecting flight to the United Kingdom and I recall waiting for my new Windows 95 installation to finish. I remember waiting outside the SoftBank shop in Ginza 4-chome, Tokyo to ensure I was one of the first people in Japan to possess the new iPhone 5 and I remember sitting in the waiting room at Koyama Driving School for my motorcycle test results. Then there was the two hour wait in the Immigration Centre in Shinagawa, Tokyo for my permanent resident visa some fourteen years earlier. I also recall waiting on a cold winter's night for enemy forces to pass by our ambush point during a military patrol exercise in the Scottish mountains and waiting for my first ever rich fruit cake to bake in the oven when I was nineteen years old. I remember a time waiting on the streets of Inverness dressed in my MacKenzie of Seaforth kilt with my platoon on a freezing cold day before marching down the main street during a Remembrance

Day parade and I remember waiting for my parents to pick me up from Belford in Northumberland after having sustained a punctured tyre on my no-spare-tyre style bicycle adventure to Haggerston Castle Holiday Park in Northumbria. There was no doubt, the golden two-hour wait award went to the motorcycle muppet lying on the E.R. table in Japan, waiting for emergency surgery.

While all this waiting was going on, the attending nurse and a medical intern did their best trying to shorten those two hours by engaging in conversation about my bike, country, time in Japan, etc.

After an hour had passed, I was wheeled off to the Radiology Department for an X-ray. When I reached the X-ray examination room, I had to be transferred manually from the wheeled stretcher and onto the radiographic table under the X-ray tube housing and that made me scream out again in pain. Every little movement brought back incredible sears of unbearable pain and I had to go through that again when I was slid back onto the trolley.

Back in the Emergency Room, Dr. Tsuchiya waited for the X-ray images to come through and asked me in the meantime if I had any known allergies. I had only one allergy I knew of and that was to penicillin. I discovered my allergy to penicillin in Newcastle General Hospital when I was thirteen years old. I had been steering a wooden cart that my friends and I had built, with my bare hands, when it hit the corner of a red brick wall and caught the flesh around the middle joint of the thumb on my right hand, known in medical terms as the proximal phallanx. I don't remember the actual allergic reaction I experienced post injection, but I doubt it was severe. In any case, the injury required ten stitches on that occasion.

When the X-ray finally came through on the E.R. computer screen, I was quite shocked at the extent of damage from what to me, initially, seemed to be a clean blow to the leg. Both lateral and anterior-posterior views clearly showed a comminuted open compound fracture of the tibia and comminuted segmental fracture of the fibula, meaning the base of both leg bones had shattered into pieces and that the tibia had pierced through the skin. There was lateral displacement of the distal tibial fragment, indicating the base of the tibia had been forced sideways out of alignment due to the impact of the bike hitting me. That explained why it was so painful. Dr. Tsuchiya admitted some two weeks later that I had presented him with the worse orthopaedic fracture case he'd ever dealt with. That certainly raised my eyebrows in this reasonably busy hospital.

The remaining hour proved an additional agonising wait as the minutes ticked slowly by, torturing me second by second. I was so relieved when the time came to go to theatre, although I started to feel some anxiety about having to have emergency surgery. Still in all my motorcycle clothing, I was taken upstairs to the operating theatre on the second floor where I donned a surgical cap and waited a short time before being trolleyed into theatre for the anaesthetist, Dr. Yanagisawa to prepare me for my trip to "paradise". She placed a soft, clear plastic oxygen mask over my face and asked me to breathe in nice and deeply. After a couple of minutes of breathing in fresh oxygen, she informed me that she had inserted a sterile hypodermic needle into the back of my hand and was administering the intravenous agent, propofol. In medical terms, this is known as the induction stage and marks the period between the initial administration of the anaesthesia agents and loss of consciousness. The second stage is known as the excitement stage and is the transition from loss of consciousness to the onset of automatic breathing. The final stage of accurate dosage of anaesthesia is referred to as the stage of surgical anaesthesia, the shift from automatic respiration to *diaphragmatic paralysis* (loss of control of one or both halves of the diaphragm caused by a traumatic injury or disease which decreases or terminates the impulse of respiratory stimuli originating in the brain).[1]

Almost immediately I felt the rush of the propofol as it quickly flowed through the veins of my body, barely counting eight seconds before I fell into a medically induced coma. Propofol is very slightly soluble in water and for that reason is used as an intravenously injectable emulsion. It is a sedative-hypnotic agent, containing 0.25 mg/mL of sodium metabisulfite and is used in both induction and maintenance of anaesthesia or sedation. Interestingly, I discovered that it also contains soybean oil, glycerol, egg yolk phospholipid and sodium hydroxide. Intravenous injection of a therapeutic dose of propofol induces hypnosis, with minimal excitation.[2] For Dr. Tsuchiya, it was time to begin surgery. For me, that brought an instant end to my pain and for what felt like a very short time, a trip to 'paradise'; a sunny deserted island somewhere in the pacific surrounded by shallow, clear blue waters, a golden sandy beach dotted with an abundance of tall coconut trees, tropical birds singing their hearts out in the background and not a single human in sight. In reality though, the time was not so short.

---

[1] *http://www.mediconotebook.com/2013/01/guedels-stages-of-anaesthesia.html*

[2] *http://www.drugs.com/pro/propofol.html*

Prior to surgery, it was obviously necessary to undress me and sterilise around the trauma site; I learned later that a theatre assistant removed my boots intact and grabbed a pair of special surgical scissors which she used to cut all the way up my motorcycle trousers and dress trousers underneath, including my underwear.

During surgery, my right foot was pulled down while my tibia was inserted back in between muscle and flesh using a special stainless steel operation room tool called a Variable Type Levator. This tool enabled the careful reinsertion of the bones without damaging the surrounding tissue. Prior to the final stages of my surgery, the anaesthetist began planning for the emergence stage which would gradually lift me out of "paradise". Physically gradual that is, but in my mind it seemed like just a few seconds, rather similar to being awoken from a deep sleep. The emergence procedure for any patient under general anaesthesia is complex and there are various options available according to the surgical procedure, like patient weight, condition of the patient, physiological status and opioid tolerance.[3] I was also administered 100% oxygen for five to ten minutes to prevent hypoxemia,

---

[3] *Manual of Clinical Anesthesiology, Larry F.Chu, Andrea J. Fuller, 2011*

oxygen deficiency in my arterial blood.[4] The operating procedure itself lasted one hundred and twenty six minutes[5] before I was transferred to a mobile bed and taken up to a room on the eighth floor of the building to recover.

It took just ten minutes from end of surgery to coming round in the room to which I was assigned. On regaining consciousness, I experienced some delirium. I recall hearing a nurse call out *"Sumisu San! Sumisu San!"* ("Mr Smyth! Mr Smyth!") which took me at least a few seconds before realising that someone was actually trying to communicate with me and was waiting for a response. When I succumbed to this new environment, I could barely move. I felt no pain but I felt quite stiff and stuck to the bed. I lay there for two hours, drifting in and out of sleep while breathing in a reduced amount of oxygen through the face mask I was still wearing.

During that time I remember the strange, somewhat intermittent feeling of involuntary urination I was experiencing. One moment, the feeling of urination, the next, that feeling gone. Then I noticed a plastic collection bag hanging off the side of the bed, one third full and a clear plastic tube running back

---

[4] *Eckman, Margaret (2010). Professional guide to pathophysiology, Wolters Kluwer/Lippincott Williams & Wilkins. p. 208*

[5] *Dr Tsuchiya confirmed time from surgery log*

under the sheets to my groin. I was wearing a *intermittent urinary catheter* (tube placed in the body to temporarily drain and collect urine from the bladder).[6] This device was of course necessary prior to emergence, perhaps even throughout surgery, but when fully conscious, it made for a rather strange feeling and was becoming quite uncomfortable, so at this stage two nurses prepared to remove it. Having a urinal catheter removed during consciousness is a wholly unpleasant experience, the details of which I shall spare you and reserve myself some dignity. Ironically, my grandmother once remarked to my mother when she was in hospital about to give birth to me that dignity is something you leave at the hospital gates and pick up again on the way out.

Now that I was awake, I could survey my leg. It was not at all painful anymore and I was once again comfortable, but I had temporarily lost all sense of time. It must have been at least five hours since my beautiful BMW had impacted my leg and forced the bone out of my skin. Although my leg was now very stiff, with all that shock and pain behind me I could focus on the most salient task of recovery. I had expected to see my leg wholly wrapped in some sort of white plaster cast (as were many of my friends who came to visit me) but I had something quite different

---

[6] *Flexible catheter used for short-term drainage of urine*

attached to my leg, from my foot right up the inside of my leg to just below my knee. I had been externally fixated.

The primary purpose of my emergency surgery was not really to orientate the bone for regrowth, although it was of course to return the bone to its correct position. My leg had been 'fixed' in order to stabilise its structure and more importantly to reduce the possibility of infection. Attached to my leg was an external skeletal fixation apparatus; a series of stainless steel bolts, adjustable clamp members and carbon fibre support rods. I'd never seen anything like this before and found it truly fascinating, so much so in fact that it was one of several aspects that inspired me to write this book.

My leg was bandaged pretty much all the way up to my knee and as I inspected the apparatus further I was surprised to see how it was actually attached to my leg. I was looking at a very clever and practical device. The apparatus had been assembled in such a way as to hold my leg in a stable position with my foot in its usual ninety degrees to my leg but making it virtually impossible for me to bend my foot to any extent. The apparatus consisted of three carbon fibre rods of varying lengths, each one attached to a multi-angle clamp member, thus practically joining the three rods together, albeit at slightly different angles. The clamps had then been attached to four 20cm long stainless steel bolts with threading extending around 10cm up the shaft. During surgery, these bolts, or pins as they are called, had been driven directly through the skin and flesh, into the bones in my leg and foot to a depth of up to 8cm. Of course, precise pre-drilling using an orthopaedic drill bit was performed prior to that to initiate smaller diameter guide holes. The first pin was securely screwed into the base of my first metatarsal bone, that is the third and largest bone of my hallux. The second pin was inserted into the *calcaneum* (largest of the tarsal bones, commonly known as the heel bone) and the remaining two pins, at 5cm apart, were securely driven right through the *periosteum* (dense layer of vascular connective tissue enveloping the bones except at the surfaces of the joints), the *cortical bone* (dense form of connective bone tissue composed chiefly of calcium salts) all the way through the marrow in the *medullary cavity* (central cavity of bone shafts where red and/or yellow bone marrow is stored), and straight out the other side.

At the base of each pin, there was a generous smear of a special antibiotic ointment called *Gentacin®*, around the exposed pin threads to create a barrier between the flesh and exterior environment. Gentacin contains the active ingredient Gentamicin Sulphate. *Gentamicin Sulphate* is the equivalent antibiotic ointment administered in the U.K. however, in the Japanese market, Gentacin is used.[7] It belongs to a class of drugs known as aminoglycoside antibiotics (bactericidal antibiotics that are effective against aerobic gram-negative bacilli and mycobacterium tuberculosis, the causative agent of most cases of tuberculosis).

For the first few days after my operation, I needed to take painkillers and Brotizolam, which is a sedative-hypnotic thienodiazepine drug (a sleeping medicine not approved for sale in the U.K.) in the late evening so that I could sleep comfortably without any pain. The apparatus attached to my leg made it extremely uncomfortable to sleep at night as I could not really lie on my side but lying through the night on my back was exceptionally uncomfortable too, given the hardness of the mattress. To alleviate the discomfort, I ended up placing a large fluffy pillow between my knees.

---

[7] *http://www.drugs.com/international/gentacin.html*

Chapter Three
Kanto Rosai

Being completely conscious of my environment now, I took time to scan the confines of the room and the space around me. I found myself in a four-person room, with a tall, light brown faux-veneered bedside cabinet to my left, a small flatscreen television securely anchored to it with a swivel mount and a pair of green and white striped cotton pajamas neatly folded on top. There was an off-white wall reading light with a 60 watt energy saving bulb in it attached to a swinging arm, a small circular gray waste paper bin labelled 'T.O.S.S.' and an adjustable bed table on casters. There was also a nurse-call handset plugged into a special socket in the wall and a spiral cable draped over the metal bed-rail close to my hand and a cream-coloured privacy curtain around the whole space. That was pretty much it. I couldn't see much else of the room or fellow patients as my neighbours had their privacy curtains drawn.

I still had no idea where I was geographically, so I grabbed my iPhone and opened the Google Maps app. Within a few seconds, I discovered I was in Kanto Rosai Hospital in the town of Motosumiyoshi, to the immediate east of Musashikosugi in Kawasaki City, and just three stops along the Toyoko Line from my local station of Tamagawa. At least I could now feel a sense of satisfaction knowing exactly where I was.

Kanto Rosai Hospital is a nine floor hospital with a fairly large footprint. To the immediate west stands a multitude of staff apartments, primarily for the nurses and younger doctors, and to the north, at the front of the building, an ample two-storey car park for the convenience of visitors, while the main building itself backs onto the Toyoko and Meguro Lines. The hospital was modernised some years ago and so it is clean, practical and reasonably well designed. Kanto Rosai is a specialist hospital for orthopaedics and sports injuries, however there is also a small maternity unit in place. On the first floor there is a Doutor brand coffee shop, with its long wooden service counter and glass refrigerated cabinet stocked with a selection of cakes and staffed by three or four people at any given time. Across from that is a small hospital convenience store, stocking a variety of snack foods, drinks, boxes of tissues, men's diapers (a term used in Japan for incontinence pads), walking sticks, soap, shampoo and other in-patient necessities. I visited both of these premises on a daily basis, once I was able to move around in a wheelchair, though I was rather disappointed to discover many of the goods in the latter were overpriced.

Within the hospital there were thirteen in-patient wards in all, two wards on each floor, all related to orthopaedics, except for the ninth floor, which had just the one ward and was used to accommodate pregnant women who were due to give birth. Each individual ward was served by a separate nurse station facing towards the other ward on the same floor, across the larger of two lift halls, with its three stainless steel-doored lifts. Each of these nurse stations was the work hub for two separate nurse teams, A Team and B Team. A Team were responsible for managing one half of the east side of the ward and B Team managed half of the west side. Each nurse station operated separately as did the two nurse teams and each nurse stayed with their respective team and nurse station. The nurse station was clinically bright and scrupulously clean. At times, a hive of activity, at other times, almost deserted. In addition to the two flat LCD monitors sitting on the beige-coloured desk at the front of each nurse station, there were at least twenty Fujitsu laptop computers around where the nurses would input and upload data. I would often see Dr. Tsuchiya there at different computer screens and sometimes his boss, Dr. Okazaki, Head of Orthopaedics. Placed against the walls were tall grey metal racks holding a myriad of paper files and a large cork-backed notice board pinned with a variety of different size notices. At the back of the station there were two large stainless steel sinks directly in front of an even larger double glazed window which overlooked Nakahara Heiwa Koen, a park founded in 1992, built in the hope for everlasting peace and featuring 'Kawasaki Peace Museum', a peace anniversary statue and an exhibit area for peace-themed sculptures. At the very front of the nurse station there usually sat a female administrator, whose job it was to deal with the day-to-day administrative requests from both patients and visitors.

Each duty nurse was responsible for serving a number of patients across several rooms who were in the same orthopaedic class, and during the course of her duties would push a waist-height trolley around with a Fujitsu laptop computer, running Windows OS, on top. All the data she would collect on each of her patients, such as medicines administered, dressings changed, intravenous catheters set up, their condition, etc., was entered into the database. Patients were even asked each day how many times they visited the toilet the previous day, or more specifically how many times they urinated and how many times they defecated.

This seemed excessive to me and often when asked this question, I would mischievously create figures from the top of my head just to break the monotony. I'd even play around with the numbers sometimes in the hope of initiating some kind of surprised reaction, which I did get from time to time. Aside from the '*number ones*' and '*number twos*', this information served not only as a report on patient history for both the nurses and doctors to access but it also served as an important administrative accounting procedure allowing the hospital Administration Department to calculate patient bills.

Given the fact that each nurse had access to the whole patient database, I was able to view my X-ray images and the tomogram images of a computed tomography (CT) scan I had some time later. This was particularly convenient for me as I was learning to read the chronographic images, analyse and closely follow the growth and development of my fractured tibia and fibula a day or so after my visits to Radiology every Thursday afternoon.

Periodically, the duty nurse would enter the room to attend to nurse calls from patients or just as part of the daily routine of checking blood pressure and temperature. I needed to call the duty nurse from time to time throughout the day to change my ice pack or to empty my plastic bottle-shaped bed pan as I was unable to leave my bed to visit the toilet for the first day or two. I was also asked to use it at night as it was not safe for me to get into my wheelchair without a nurse present and visit the toilet unassisted.

In the first ward room in which I stayed, no-one really spoke to me, aside from the usual "*Ohayougozaimasu*", meaning "Good Morning". Had I not initiated those words to the man in the bed space directly across from mine, I am sure he wouldn't even have eye-balled me, which to be honest, he really didn't do anyway. Of course I was primarily focused on my recovery but I couldn't help but feel somewhat isolated and socially deprived which can prove to be rather demotivating for someone who is socially and business-wise, an excellent communicator. Although I have difficulty some of the time with my Japanese comprehension, I am more than capable of holding a conversation in Japanese, but it's very tiresome to continually generate questions instead of wholly interacting with the other party, which is the normal business of dialogue. Sometimes I really feel I am justifying that wonderful English idiomatic expression "*flogging a dead horse*".

Japanese society is renowned for its first class quality in service and production, a fact for which I have absolutely no argument and in which I endlessly relish. There is an all round degree of politeness and respect among the population. Japan is a passive country with a deep sense of peace and caring for others. It's a democratic economy with a stable political system and, with few exceptions, a country any foreigner can feel safe in, but what it is *not* is a country renowned for its great social cohesion.

Tokyo, with a population of twenty million people, was deemed the "smartest" city in the world according to a study published earlier in 2014, 'IESE Cities in Motion Indices 2014', conducted by the IESE School of Business at the University of Navarra in Barcelona. The ranking was based along ten different dimensions to determine efficiency. Tokyo was deemed best for 'human capital', meaning that it should be able to attract and retain talent, create plans to improve education and boost creativity and research. However, perhaps not surprisingly, Tokyo was ranked 125th for social cohesion.[8]

Barely a week had gone by when I was asked to move to another room on the same floor but on the west side of the building. In the room I had been using, I had an obstructed outside view as there was a reasonable sized fridge in front of the window. In contrast, the new bed-space I was moving into was right alongside the window and I was afforded a glorious view of Motosumiyoshi and the tip of the

---

[8] *IESE Cities in Motion Indice 2014*

Yokohama skyline. I could just about make out Landmark Tower, the icon of Yokohama. The downside was that there was no fridge available in this room but I was rewarded with a decent view as the room I was in was on the eighth floor.

In this new room, my neighbours were a little more forthcoming with their communication, after some prompting from me of course. The young Japanese man directly across from me, *Kota Yamada*, was friendly enough and always exchanged morning and evening greetings but at the same time shrouded his bed space with the curtains which I soon labelled '*conversation killers*'. The sliding doors to each room were always open during the day and often through the night so on passing I observed to my amazement that most people had their '*conversation killers*' drawn.

My newly-acquired room-mate, Kota, warmed up to conversation the more I spoke to him, particularly when a new patient arrived to move into my former neighbour's bed space. Kota had been involved in a motorcycle accident a couple of months previously and was diagnosed with Compartment Syndrome, which occurs when excessive pressure builds up inside an enclosed space in the body. Compartment syndrome usually results from bleeding or swelling after an injury. The dangerously high pressure in compartment syndrome impedes the flow of blood to and from the affected tissues.[9] In Kota's case, it was an emergency, requiring surgery to prevent permanent injury. Kota was not a particularly outstanding man with regard to his physical build or his appearance but the first thing that drew my attention was that he had a peculiar and cumbersome-looking apparatus around his leg. I thought until this point that my external fixation device was quite complex, but Kota's external apparatus was more complicated looking than mine and occupied a full 360 degree radius around his leg. It was composed of several metal rings, cables, dampers and adjusters. What's more, his apparatus had a special name, it was called the *Ilizarov Apparatus*. At the time, I knew absolutely nothing about this equipment but I would soon learn much. I later discovered that several people in the hospital wore the Ilizarov Apparatus, each assembled differently according to their medical condition and osteosynthetic needs. This was not just an orthopaedic hospital but as I was soon to learn, it was one of the best orthopaedic hospitals in Japan.

The Ilizarov Apparatus was invented by Dr. Gavriil Abramovich Ilizarov, a Russian Orthopaedic Surgeon, and former engineer whose only formal surgical training had been a six month course in military field surgery. Dr. Ilizarov first became interested in

---

[9] *http://www.webmd.com/pain-management/guide/compartment-syndrome-causes-treatments*

orthopaedics and bone reconstruction because many of his patients were soldiers returning from the front line battles of World War II, many of whom suffered severe fractures. As for Dr. Ilizarov's device itself, the following extract from a paper by a student doctor from Oxford University Hospitals NHS Trust clearly describes the apparatus:

> *The Ilizarov apparatus is a set of external fixators consisting of rings, rods and kirschner wires, all made of stainless steel. It differs from the conventional external fixators in that it encases the limb as a cylinder and it uses wires instead of pins to fix the bone to the rings. The circular construction and tensioned wires allow early weight bearing as it provides far greater support than monolateral (one sided) fixators. The top rings of the Ilizarov fixator allow force to be transferred through the external frame, bypassing the fracture site and transferring the force from healthy bone to healthy bone.*
>
> *The purpose of the Ilizarov fixator is to stimulate bone growth, and this works by the principle of distraction osteogenesis, which is the*

> *pulling apart of bone to stimulate new bone growth.*[10]

In 1951, Dr. Ilizarov proposed his own device for bone fracture consolidation which eventually resulted in the development of a new scientific and practical trend in the field of orthopaedics, later named 'compression distraction osteosynthesis'. In 1971, Dr. Ilizarov was appointed Director of the *Kurgan Research Institute for Experimental and Clinical Orthopaedics and Traumatology.*

The method of compression distraction osteosynthesis offered orthopaedic surgeons around the world a greater study into the biology of tissue regeneration in general, and into the theory of bone formation in particular. After the split of the USSR in 1991, Dr. Ilizarov became Director General of the Russian Scientific Center for Restorative Traumatology and Orthopaedics in Kurgan but passed away the following year, on 24th July, 1992.[11]

For the first couple of weeks I got to know the elderly man to my left and although he was a little reserved at first to say much to me, it wasn't long before he became sufficiently relaxed to want to talk

---

[10] *http://www.ouh.nhs.uk/limbreconstruction/information/documents/Ilizarovtechniqueforlimbreconstruction.pdf*

[11] *http://www.ilizarov.ru/en/index.php?option=com_content&view=article&id=315*

constantly. I understood what he was saying most of the time but it became difficult for me when he muttered or spoke excitedly at high speed. However, both he, and his wife who visited frequently, were a very pleasant and friendly couple and I was happy to have met them. However, he sported, without fail, an incessant desire to break wind from behind the curtain. Between the wind would come the burps right after each mealtime and then when brushing his teeth he'd regurgitate like a farmyard animal or a cat having difficulty trying to cough up a fur-ball. I've no doubt this was all part of his medical problem but it wasn't a pleasant experience for those within earshot. One day, he noticed me sketching a copy of a photograph I had taken of part of Braemar in Scotland and became quite ecstatic about it, so on the day he was discharged I presented him with the sketch. He was so elated and I was so relieved to be free of listening to his bodily noises.

The older gentleman in the space diagonally from me didn't really say anything other than the usual morning greetings. Then, one day when I was sketching in my bed, he suddenly called across to me and started speaking in English. I was a bit taken aback but nevertheless delighted to satisfy his desire to have a little conversation with me in English. All this time he had been silent and then suddenly he had decided to speak in English which really took me by surprise. However, I later discovered that he had been planning for a few days to speak to me but wanted to collect an adequate number of phrases and vocabulary before he plucked up sufficient courage to start the engine of dialogue, based on the notes he'd taken. He'd understand and anticipate some of the answers I gave him but then I would try to expand upon my answer and he would quickly move on to the next question.

The social cohesion in our room was about to improve though when two new patients arrived just after the old man diagonally across from me was discharged. One of them was totally alert and sitting upright, the other was lying down, almost lifeless. To my left was a small, somewhat short, stalky twenty seven year old man with whom I quickly formed a good rapport. His name was *Ryuji Maeguchi*. Ryuji had the grave misfortune to have fractured the navicular and cuboid bones on his right foot and in doing so had simultaneously separated the entire phalange range from the normally connected metatarsal range on his left foot, meaning his toes were basically separated due to the impact of a four metre fall from a communications tower on which he was working. For a while, he was bound to the wheelchair he was using and only started to use crutches a few days before I checked out.

Ryuji, my other hospital friend, Kota and I got on well and had a good laugh and chat until the night duty nurse came around at 9:00pm each night to say good night and switch the lights off; however, this didn't stop us as we would still continue to chat well after that. When Kota was discharged a couple of weeks later, Ryuji was left with the challenge of understanding my often strange explanations in Japanese, explanations of things I wanted to discuss. As a consequence of the situation, I had inadvertently sparked a desire in him to learn English, which was a big challenge for him as he was almost incapable of speaking or understanding a word of my native language. He was highly motivated though and began to make notes on the vocabulary I translated for him. Soon, he was able to understand some of the things I was saying in English.

The old man across from Ryuji was incomprehensible and the only sounds which he emitted were grunts of aggression when he wanted the attention of the nursing staff. Most of the time this turned out to be of no real necessity and simply impinged on the nurses' more pressing duties. Other times, we witnessed the discomfort and personal agony the old man was experiencing as a result of his double incontinence and it soon became evident, he was in dire need of help.

On many occasions, for all in that small ward, as well as the poor patient himself, it was a very unpleasant experience. Due to my restricted mobility it was impossible to make a quick exit from this small ward and I had therefore to endure the extremely odeous gases coming from the direction of the old man's bed - smells which left the other patients and myself nauseated. However, as much as I felt compassion for this patient's predicament the only help I could offer was to summon the nurses who had the unpleasant job of dealing with the situation. Until that time I hadn't realised he was so ill and just thought he wanted to sleep most of the time through the day and when awake, had no desire to be sociable. It became clear to me that he was not only suffering as a result of a general medical illness but that he was suffering from some form of dementia, hence his inability to behave in a normal way. When I went over next day to see if he was feeling better I observed that he was almost skeletal and was clearly a very sick old man, unaware of where he was and what was happening to him. On his shrunken face he wore a lifeless expression and it was evident he was unable to communicate socially. Much of the time he would just lie there open-mouthed, staring blankly across the room and frequently he would call out loudly for the nurses' attention with a gruff *"Ne!"*, a rough translation of *"Hey!"*; not the politest way of seeking assistance.

I noticed he was intravenously fed liquid food and water from 500ml packs hanging from the I.V. hook apparatus attached to the ceiling. I googled his intravenous food nutrient pack and found it was extremely expensive, at ¥7,000 (approx. $64) per 500ml bag. It may well have cost eight times the price of my meals but I'm pretty sure it didn't taste like a big juicy, succulent sirloin steak grill-charred with French peppercorns, served with sautéed fresh chanterelle mushrooms in a Bordeaux red wine sauce, with a side dish of fluffy dauphinoise potatoes blended with a generous amount of fresh double cream, oven roasted thyme and nut potatoes, shallot, tomato and dill stuffed bell peppers and delicate smoke steamed aubergines. Then again, neither did mine.

The elderly patient's incessant shouts were so bad that every night, around 11:00pm, he would be wheeled out of the room and placed in the lift hall in front of the nurse station. That meant that while everyone else could now hear him, back in our room we were at least afforded a significant decrease in volume. His wife would visit him almost every day, each time apologising to us for the noise he reportedly made in her absence, and prompting us to agree that he was noisy and annoying. Of course, our response to her was *"no, no, not at all, it's okay, don't worry about it"*, all the time praying she'd have him moved and give us peace.

I became friendly with many people in the hospital, particularly those I had met in the ward or rehabilitation gym and now enjoy keeping in touch with them through social media. Shortly after I was moved, for the third time to a new room, I became friends with a young Japanese patient whose name was *Takeo Okubo*. Unfortunately Takeo San couldn't speak a word of English but was nevertheless a very good communicator and we could understand each other quite well. He was a good listener and could interpret my sometimes rather strange or grammatically incorrect Japanese sentences. Takeo San was in his early thirties, around 170cm tall and of a fairly strong physique. I learned that he was in the construction business and had had an operation on his knee due to a fall he had at work, whilst carrying several sheets of plasterboard. Although he was physically strong on the outside and confident in character I soon discovered he was also very caring and exceptionally kind-hearted. Takeo was one of the nicest persons I had met for a long time. He was always polite, appreciative and extremely considerate towards others. He made friends with many other patients and once discharged from the hospital would make a point of visiting them each time he returned for his weekly out-patient rehabilitation sessions.

Takeo was one of two new friends with whom I got on particularly well. The other was a man whom I first heard talking and laughing in the hallway, outside his room. His voice made me curious enough to get off my bed late one morning whilst I was in the middle of composing an e-mail to my mother, don my slippers, grab my crutches and see who this fellow was, for although he was speaking Japanese at native level, he laughed like I had never heard any Japanese man laugh. He was laughing practically every thirty seconds and I could hear the nurses he was chatting with were laughing too. As I stepped out of my room into the corridor, I could see that he appeared to be a jolly person of mixed race. Immediately we greeted each other in Japanese and he confirmed he was indeed half Japanese and half Iranian. His father was Iranian and his mother Japanese. He had been in Japan for twenty three years and in Kanto Rosai for three weeks due to an operation he had on his back, stemming from an accident he had in his renovation business. Although able to stand upright without nurse assistance, I noticed he required a special walking frame for support, although a few weeks after my discharge, he was able to walk with the aid of two walking sticks.

He had introduced himself as *Tora Andy*. Tora was fifty years old but didn't look a day over forty. He was good looking and almost as tall as I, at around 184cm. With his short brown hair, well trimmed beard, lively personality and his stature, he looked very striking. It was easy to understand why the nurses enjoyed his company and were like *'bees round the honey pot'*. Without doubt, he was one of the cheeriest fellows in the hospital and with his excellent Japanese language skills was able to do what I *would* have done if I *could* have but ... *didn't!* He was able to chat to anyone he came across and share his great sense of humour, generating a feeling of well-being in almost everyone he met.

So Tora and I hit it off immediately, both sharing a great sense of humour and both having lived in Japan for a similar length of time with an equal in-depth understanding of Japanese culture. What was even more pleasing to me was that in addition to his Japanese and Persian language skills, he could also speak fluent English. Now, I had found someone to chat to about anything and everything and so we did, every day. He would come to my room, I would visit the room he was in, or we'd be found chatting to other patients or nurses in the corridor. A couple of weeks before I was discharged, we made it a routine to visit the cafe on the first floor after the rehabilitation sessions, sometimes joined by some other friends we made there.

Although Tora had absolutely no problem communicating in Japanese with anyone, whether staff, other patients or visitors, he was obviously delighted to make friends with another foreigner. Together, we'd try to brighten everyone's day. We always made people laugh and that was definitely good for health.

A couple of weeks later, Tora's doctor suggested he move to the seventh floor as there was an empty room there and a bed that was more suitable for his back, so we resorted to using LINE to communicate and arrange to meet in the cafe downstairs.

When I was not chatting to people, I would be emailing, browsing the net or researching medical journals whilst hitching a ride on the wifi tethering capability of my iPhone. When Tora was not chatting to people, almost a rare occasion, he'd be as surrounded by technology as I was, only instead of researching, he would be keeping a watchful eye on his Forex trading platform, performing online trades from time to time. I had planned on doing the same on my NYSE trading platform but my internet speed was slower in the evenings, when the stock market was open. Tora was using a mobile wifi router with better speed. Instead, I decided to write a book, which I hope

Tora will buy with the money he gained from his Forex trading!

Aside from the odd snacks I'd have in the cafe or the snacks I bought in the hospital shop, I relied on the meals served three times a day. Hospital meals arrived in individual small dishes sitting on a brown molded plastic tray. They were fairly insignificant on the whole and it was fish that was mostly to be found on the menu. Each meal included a large bowl of steamed rice. Without fail, breakfast consisted of a bowl of steamed rice, a bowl of miso soup and a small dish containing some pickled vegetables. I never once touched the pickled vegetables which were served with *every* meal and although I ate the rice, it was becoming incredibly boring and I quickly began to lose my appetite for it. For a man who pretty much throughout his entire life has enjoyed continental style breakfasts consisting of a bowl of tasty cereal or muesli with fresh pasteurised milk, a glass of cold fresh orange juice, a tub of creamy yoghurt, a slice or two of hot toasted bread with butter and a variety of preserves all washed down with a mug of steaming hot tea, facing a tray of rice, miso soup with seaweed and cold brain-crunching pickles was not in the least bit appetising. Nevertheless it *was* food, and to make it at least sound more appealing, I thought of breakfasts as more of a tray of nutrients necessary for my leg's regeneration.

Lunch was always 170 grams of either fish, pork, chicken, fish again or more fish, served with a bowl of rice and some pickles. Dinner was simply hit or miss for me. Sometimes a decent piece of chicken breast, or pork tonkatsu would appear, but more often than not, fish would be lying under the plastic dish cover. I didn't realise until the beginning of August that it was actually possible to choose between two meal sets for breakfast and dinner, Set A and Set B. I was now able to reduce the percentage of fish for dinner by almost half and I could choose set B, a "bread set" for breakfast. The "bread set" consisted of hot watery soup with either pieces of egg swimming in it or slices of seaweed, sometimes both, a cold slice of solidified scrambled egg without seasoning, two slices of warm bread sealed in a plastic bag and a single serving of jam, likewise presented in a small plastic bag. I supplemented my breakfasts with some items from the hospital shop and so every morning in August, I had a hot cup of fresh coffee, courtesy of my small Nespresso coffee machine, and one big jam and banana sandwich. I never tired of that breakfast. If it hadn't been for the fruit, bread, ice-cream, chocolate and snacks in the hospital convenience store, I'd probably have gone '*nuts*'!

One of the more positive things about the meals though was that sometimes a small piece of fruit in syrup, sealed in a single portion bag would be on the tray. Towards the end of my stay in hospital, I saved each of these little fruit bags in the equally tiny refrigerator I was renting and the day before I was discharged, I made a large half kilogram fruit salad, topped with strawberry yoghurt from the overpriced hospital shop. *Delicious!*

Aside from the unappetising food, this was a reasonably good hospital to stay in although I have never actually stayed in a hospital in the U.K., or any other country for that matter so it is perhaps hard to judge. However, Kanto Rosai was not the only hospital in *Japan* where I had been an in-patient.

Chapter Four
Kechouen

On the evening of Christmas Day 2008, an ambulance arrived at the house to rush me to Denen Central Hospital, about a five minute journey from home. I was in agony with a very dull pain in my abdomen. It felt as though I had been kicked in the stomach by an entire football team. I was convinced it was food poisoning. Less than two hours earlier, my wife, Noriko and I had been in a restaurant not far from home and now, on reflection, (despite my knowledge of its change of ownership), I began to question my sanity at having gone back to the same restaurant which had resulted in my contracting food poisoning some ten years earlier.

In 1998 I had gone to that restaurant for a meal and had suffered salmonella food poisoning as a result of consuming undercooked chicken breast. I became violently ill and was taken to hospital and diagnosed with food poisoning as a direct result of the restaurant's poor food preparation. The experience was so drastic, it knocked me out for a whole week, though as it transpired, this time round in 2008, the problem was *not* the fault of the restaurant's food preparation. However, the diagnosis in hospital revealed something quite unexpected.

Just a few days prior, I had contracted a lower respiratory tract infection. Not surprising as I frequently commuted by crowded train and had witnessed many of the passengers coughing and sneezing while many others wore face masks. Cold and flu viruses are almost unavoidable if you travel by train in Tokyo, especially in the Winter months. At the time of the initial symptoms, I visited the family doctor to confirm my own diagnosis and was prescribed a course of fluoroquinolone-based antibiotics, a class of synthetic broad-spectrum antibacterial drugs, which for the first few days seemed to be working, but trouble was just around the corner - big trouble.

For the first couple of days I completely lost my appetite, but soon began to recover and felt like eating a reasonably hearty meal, so my family and I decided to visit the aforementioned restaurant. I ordered a side dish of French fries with my meal and devoured every last morsel. Things seemed good and I was happy to be recovering well from the virus.

We walked back home from the restaurant and my wife left in the car with my daughter to visit her mother, about ten minutes drive away. I decided to stay home. Less than an hour later, I started to experience an uncomfortable feeling in my stomach and then a dull pain. I thought it would reach a peak and then subside, but it just kept getting worse. It became so uncomfortable, that I lay on the floor, groaning and hoping it would stop. It reached the point where I lay curled up on the floor in utter pain when I called Noriko and asked her to quickly come and pick me up, but instead, she wisely called an ambulance, so I forced myself up, grabbed my wallet, donned my jacket and shoes and locked the front door behind me. I struggled to the bottom of the tiled steps and waited for the ambulance, clenching my stomach and holding back the need to groan out loud now that I was in front of the house.

A few minutes later, the ambulance with siren I had heard blaring from several blocks away, now silenced, arrived. As the tailgate opened, I climbed in and lay down on the trolley. At that point Noriko arrived and followed the ambulance to the hospital.

Christmas Day was a Thursday and the hospital was closed in the evening except for emergencies so it took a little while for the duty doctor to attend to me. When he arrived, I was lying down on the trolley in the small emergency room holding on to my stomach in the hope that the incredible dull pain would subside. The doctor, a young man in his late twenties attended to me. He didn't speak a word of English so I needed to converse in Japanese but I wasn't exactly in the mood to switch on my Japanese language skills as my mind was totally fixed on the pain. He immediately hooked me up to an intravenous pain killing drug, while I groaned for its efficacy to kick in. I had never felt such deep, dull pain before.

Around an hour after the doctor had initially administered the pain killer, still shaken, I could at least sit upright again. I rested like that for another hour or so before I felt fit enough to return home. However, given my symptoms, the doctor arranged for me to return to the hospital the next morning and prepare to stay for a few days so I could be closely monitored.

Denen Central Hospital is a small hospital directly across from Den-en-chofu Station in Ota Ward, south western Tokyo. It was an old, square building that seemed to have survived for a few decades unchanged. It had no real E.R. entrance. Ambulances would just pull up right at the front entrance where everyone who visited the hospital would enter, and any casualty would then be rushed past members of the public to the attendance room to be given emergency treatment.

The next morning, I arrived at the hospital around 08:00am with some spare clothes, wash kit, towels, shaver, a book and my laptop computer. After checking-in, I was taken upstairs to the third floor and to the room I was to be in for the next four days. It was a very small room with four beds. The curtains were drawn around the other beds, so I couldn't see if there were any other patients in the room, but I suspected there were. There was a small side unit next to the bed and a hospital bed table, but nothing else. When I settled in, a nurse came to set up an intravenous catheter in my arm connected to a saline drip. I was on this drip for the first forty eight hours. During that time, I wasn't allowed to eat or drink anything other than *Pocari Sweat,* the Japanese sports drink created by the Japanese Pharmaceuticals company, Otsuka.

Pocari Sweat has a certain off-putting or humorous connotation for native English speaking markets though has an interesting history. It was developed in 1973, by one of the company's researchers who noticed a doctor drinking an I.V. solution after surgery to rehydrate himself. This gave him the idea for a potable I.V. solution. So Otsuka set out to develop a beverage that could replenish the body's water and electrolytes lost whilst sweating. The word *pocari* itself has no specified meaning.[12]

---

[12] *https://www.otsuka.co.jp/en/company/business/rehydration/pocarisweat/*

By day two, I was very hungry but had to wait until the following day before I could have any solids. When day three arrived, a breakfast tray was brought to my bed. This was my first introduction to solids since admittance to the hospital. Not quite my usual continental style of yoghurt, cereal, bread, fruit and coffee but a bowl of what looked like watery porridge, only porridge would have been somewhat tastier. It certainly lacked seasoning but I was grateful for any nutrients that could be introduced into my body at the time. By the next day, I was still on this *'porridge'* but it had become somewhat more solid and together with soft vegetables resembling steamed pumpkin and potato, I was slowly being introduced to normal food again. On the last day, I remember being served some chicken and rice and feeling much better for that.

It was only four days but it seemed such a long time, partly because I had never stayed in hospital before and I was away from my normal environment but mostly because I was not allowed to use my computer in the room with wi-fi. Without being online, I felt totally disconnected from the outside world. From this small alien world, I was temporarily unable to browse the internet, download and respond to mail, or watch videos. Moreover, I couldn't communicate live with my family and friends. My parents were worried about me and I wanted to be in Skype communication with them. I decided to walk, together with my mobile intravenous pole, to the small day room that overlooked the station hoping to find a suitable connection but it was all to no avail. In any case, long days as they were, I knew I would be released soon and I looked forward to that time. I was unable to contact my friends so easily and besides, it was a little too short notice for them to visit me, so consequently, apart from my wife and daughter, I had no visitors.

The doctor I was assigned to was unable to speak any English, as were any of the nurses or other staff. His medical explanations of my symptoms and cause were frustratingly incomprehensible and it didn't seem to register with him that I just didn't understand what was going on inside my body. Many of the Japanese medical terms he used probably wouldn't have made sense to anyone outside the medical profession anyway, so there was only one solution, given the fact that I had no access to the internet to do any research. I asked Noriko to bring me one of my human biology books[13] from home, and I spent some time trying to digest the appropriate information in it to make some sense of what was happening to me. When I was sure I understood, I presented the appropriate diagrams to the doctor and translated the textual entries into

---

[13] *"Advanced Biology" - Nelson Publishing - Michael Roberts, Michael Reiss, Grace Monger, 2000*

Japanese as best I could. He confirmed the details in my notes as accurate and finally I understood what was wrong with me, and what had caused my abdominal pain.

I was surprised to learn that as a result of the antibiotics I had been prescribed for my lower respiratory tract infection, I had contracted Clostridium Difficile Colitis, a bacterial infection. Some particular antibiotics like penicillin, cephalosporins and fluoroquinolones can interfere with the natural balance of normal bacteria in the gut that protects against clostridium difficile infection. This in turn had affected my digestive system.

From my recent biology study, I learned that during the process of digestion, a synthesised form of cholesterol is produced by the liver and in turn that cholesterol synthesises bile salts which play an important part in digestion by emulsifying fats in the small intestine. The cholesterol is synthesised by a metabolic pathway that leads from acetyl coenzyme, after which any excess cholesterol is excreted in the bile. The amount of cholesterol in the blood is determined for the most part by the type of food consumed, in conjunction with the metabolic activities of the liver. Excess cholesterol elimination constitutes an important function of the liver.

There are two sodium bile salts that are produced by the liver and form part of the bile, namely sodium taurocholate and sodium glycocholate. These two salts in the bile are stored in the gall bladder before being released into the bile duct and into the duodenum. The primary role of these two sodium bile salts is to emulsify fats by lowering their surface tension, resulting in a breakdown into numerous tiny droplets. As a result of this action, the digestive action of the enzyme lipase is facilitated as the total surface area of the fat is increased. In my body, the clostridium difficile colitis infection was slowing down the action of the sodium salts in my gall bladder. Any fats that entered my oesophagus and partly digested by the action of hydrochloric acid in my stomach would end up having trouble being broken down further in my gall bladder by the bile salts and consequently, the lipase enzyme would be unable to perform the action of digestion fast enough. This overload was what was causing the immense dull pain I had experienced, and that fat had come from the French fries I had consumed in the family restaurant.

I was relieved when I was able to leave hospital. Over the weeks following my discharge, I had to be really careful about the food I was eating not least for the fact I dreaded ever having to stay in a hospital again.

Chapter Five
Osteosythesis

Following my motorcycle accident on 5th June 2014, the objective of my initial emergency operation in Kanto Rosai Hospital had been to simply wash out the site of injury, return and reset my tibia and fibula, close the wound and stabilise my leg to ensure the elimination of any infection. However, shortly after, I would need to go through another operation. This second operation was very important and had a far greater impact on my health than I could ever have imagined. The objective for the second operation was to complete the first stage of my osteosynthesis, the surgical procedure that would stabilise and help join the ends of my fractured tibia through the use of a metal rod and a few screws.

However, although surgery was both essential and planned, it could not be executed until a certain medical criteria had been satisfied. Given the trauma my leg had gone through, the tissue surrounding the fracture was suffering from inflammation alongside its fight against infection. This is where the Head of Orthopaedics, Dr. Okazaki, got involved.

Dr. Okazaki was a fairly tall man, around 183cm in height, had a very closely trimmed head of hair and very assertive character which clearly defined his authority. He was nevertheless approachable and very helpful in explaining to me the complexities of my blood chemistry. In the process, he presented me with a hard copy of my blood chemistry, in Japanese, explaining in English that this inflammation was triggering my liver into synthesising higher levels of C-Reactive protein (CRP), an annular (ring-shaped), pentameric protein present in my blood plasma, the levels of which were rising in response to the inflammation at the base of my leg. He told me the blood samples taken from me since June 6th had been subject to a CRP test that would measure the amount of CRP in my blood plasma. He explained to me that the test was not so accurate and couldn't show where the inflammation itself was located. Instead, it could only measure general levels of inflammation in my body.

From research I conducted later, I discovered that C-Reactive protein, discovered by Tillett and Francis in 1930, binds itself to the phosphocholine on the surface of dead or dying cells, which in turn activates the compliment system, thus promoting phagocytosis by macrophages, which clears necrotic and apoptotic cells and bacteria. In the case of my trauma, the tissue injury and cell necrosis caused the release of interleukin-6 and other cytokines that triggered the synthesis of CRP and fibrinogen by the liver. CRP levels normally rise within two to six hours of surgery, up to 50,000-fold, and then go down by the third day after surgery. If CRP levels stay elevated three days after surgery, an infection may be present. Apart from liver failure, there are few known factors that interfere with CRP production.[14]

From the information Dr. Okazaki handed me, I could see that my CRP levels were listed across the period 6-11 June, representing five separate blood samples from different days. He informed me that at the current level, Dr. Tsuchiya would not be able to perform the planned surgical procedure to insert an intramedullary rod through the centre of my tibia. If my CRP levels did not drop to at least 2.0mg/dL, I would have to have a preliminary operation to re-open the trauma site and flush out the area in order to eliminate any infection and reduce the inflammation, and furthermore, I was up against the clock. A blood sample needed to be taken again on Wednesday 11th June and if that did not show decreased levels of CRP then the deciding factor between two different surgical

[14] *"C-reactive protein: a critical update". J. Clin. Invest., 2003 111 (12): 1805–12*

procedures would be determined just two days later on Friday 13th June.

When Friday arrived and I had that final, determining blood sample taken at 07:04am, I had to experience another wait of uncertainty. It was of course the weekend and I wouldn't receive the results from Dr. Okazaki until Monday morning, the actual day of my operation. When Monday finally arrived, Dr. Okazaki came in to see me around 07:30am. Amazingly, as if on cue, my CRP levels had dropped to 0.84mg/dL. I felt a mixture of relief and a slight sense of anxiety. I was now about to undergo the planned intramedullary surgery.

About an hour or so later, I was presented with a theatre gown and a cap and shortly after that was wheel-chaired into one of the large lifts and taken down to the operating theatre on the second floor.

On entering the operation rooms' area on the other side of the metal fire doors, the atmosphere had clearly moved up a few notches on the clinical scale. The first room, a pre-operation preparation room was spacious and clean. In this area, I had to don my surgical cap before continuing through an automated sliding glass door which led eventually into a wide corridor with several operating theatres on the left side. Being taken into an area where another human being is about to slice right into your flesh and drill a hole down into your bones would probably not prove to be the most comfortable moment for the majority of people, but I was quite confident, perhaps even a little excited about being there.

I was wheeled into one of these rooms and immediately met with the anaesthetist, Dr. Zaitsu, who greeted me in English and asked if he could practise his English on me. How could I possibly refuse a man who is about to stick a needle in the back of my hand and place me in a coma as I am connected to a machine that, if switched off, I would die? I didn't need to think too hard on that one anyway as his English was very good and he had a very motivated interest in improving his ability to communicate with English patients. We chatted about the procedures involved in preparing me for surgery. I watched him prepare the anaesthetic equipment and drugs and he answered my questions enthusiastically. He explained what some of the equipment was for and briefed me on the anaesthetic procedure for my surgery. Once again I would be administered, by mask induction, a carefully calculated amount of that amazing anaesthetic drug that contains soybean oil, glycerol, egg yolk phospholipid and sodium hydroxide, in order to introduce my body to a coma. The propofol was accompanied by an injection of 5ml Rocuronium Bromide, an amino steroid neuromuscular blocker.

This muscle relaxant was used to facilitate endotracheal intubation and to provide skeletal muscle relaxation during my surgery and mechanical ventilation.

In addition to the propofol, I was also administered sevoflurane, a sweet-smelling, highly fluorinated methyl isopropyl ether, nonflammable and nonexplosive liquid muscle relaxant, administered by vaporization, which works by depressing activity in the central nervous system, causing loss of consciousness.[15] The anaesthetic's name derives from having seven fluorine atoms in its substituents, together with a standard suffix for such agents. Sevoflurane, apparently, is the preferred agent for mask induction due to its lesser irritation to mucous membranes.[16] Sevoflurane was discovered by Dr. Ross C. Terrell, a pioneer in fluorinated anaesthetics research and modern anaesthesia.[17] Dr. Terrell was regarded as one of the world's leading fluorine chemists and the father of modern safe inhalation anaesthetic agents. Interestingly, Dr. Terrell has in fact synthesized most of the inhalation anaesthetics used today, including desflurane, enflurane, isoflurane, and

---

[15] *http://www.drugs.com/pro/sevoflurane.html*

[16] *http://www.sigmaaldrich.com/analytical-chromatography/air-monitoring/applications/anesthetic-gases.html*

[17] *http://www.cas.ca/English/Ross-Terrell*

sevoflurane.[18] First reports on the use of sevoflurane appeared in literature in 1971. It was introduced into clinical practice initially in Japan in 1990 and I was about to experience its effects.

The minimum alveolar concentration (MAC) of Sevoflurane in oxygen for an adult my age is 2.1%. I was administered the agent in a mixture of nitrous oxide and oxygen for approximately sixty seconds.

The first stage in my operation was to shave my reasonably hairy legs after which the external fixation apparatus bolted to my first metatarsal, calcaneum and tibia was disassembled and removed. This involved loosening the black 8mm hex-head nuts on the hinge clamps and removing both 15mm diameter carbon fibre rods and metal clamps to leave just the four 8mm diameter pins. The pins were then unscrewed from the aforementioned bones. After removal of these pins, my leg was washed with a surgical scrub called povidone-iodine, a stable chemical complex of elemental iodine and polyvinylpyrrolidone to prevent any infection. Thereafter, a surgical leg support was placed under my knees to raise my leg and orientate the top of my tibia for ease of access. When Dr. Tsuchiya was ready to proceed with the surgery, he reportedly took a scalpel and made a 4cm longitudinal incision at the base of my knee while my skin and the surrounding flesh was

---

[18] *http://www.ncbi.nlm.nih.gov/pubmed/21642612*

held apart with two surgical retracting tools. The patellar tendon was then split vertically with the scalpel in order to access the tibial plateau. A surgical orthopaedic awl was then used to enlarge the hole in my tibia, through the anterior intercondylar area and into the intramedullary space and a guide wire inserted into the tibial shaft.

The next procedure was to place an intramedullary nail over the guide wire and hammer the nail into the tibial shaft and across the fracture site. Two separate incisions were then made and proximal locking screws were placed through my tibia and nail, locking it in place. Further incisions were made at the distal end of the tibia to insert another three locking screws. When the procedure was complete, the retractors were removed and the wound and incisions were closed with polydioxanone synthetic sutures.

During the emergence stage, Dr. Zaitsu removed the endotracheal tube from my trachea, and I was given 100% oxygen for ten minutes via mask inhalation. I was then transferred to my bed and taken back to the eighth floor, where I continued on a reduced amount of oxygen from a short, black oxygen bottle. The gap between my emergence time and orientation time was relatively short but I felt utterly exhausted. Post-anaesthesia, the time when I was actually conscious and aware of my environment, I fell into normal sleep.

Two hours later, I was taken off oxygen assistance and the mask was removed. I noticed once again that I was wearing a urinal catheter. At least I knew what to expect, as if that was any comfort. With that observation out of the way, I focused on my leg condition. Although I was able to raise the bed angle to sit slightly off the horizontal, I couldn't move my leg. No matter how much I strained, I barely managed a few centimetres. This leg, wrapped in a bandage now, from my ankle to my knee, was going to take some time to rehabilitate.

Each day, for the first week or so, Dr. Tsuchiya, with the assistance of a nurse, would inspect and change my dressings. The first time he removed the partly blood soaked bandage, my leg really didn't look like it belonged to me. It looked like an alien object covered in a mix of dried povidone-iodine and blood, with several sutures on the incision areas as well as the primary trauma wound. I snapped some pictures with my iPhone camera and Dr. Tsuchiya did exactly the same with his iPhone. The dressings were a blooded mess and were duly discarded into a clear polythene bag.

A few days later, when the bandages were removed, the leg appeared in a cleaner state but post-operative bruising was clearly evident. Given the trauma my leg had just gone through, this was not a surprise. The bleeding had reduced significantly and my leg and I yearned for a proper wash. At that stage, I hadn't had a shower for almost a week but had of course been given a thorough, hot, wet, toweling down on my bed by two nurses on a daily basis over the next few days. As each new day passed I gained strength and was able to wash myself with the assistance of the nurse who would continue to towel-wash my right leg between showers. Gradually, as I gained more confidence, the nurse would hand me a bag of steaming hot towels to complete the job myself. It was nice to be able to clean myself down with hot towels but they were no substitute for a shower. I needed a shower and longed for a proper shampoo. I had been using dry shampoo everyday for the past week and as it contained alcohol, it was starting to irritate my scalp. The last thing I needed was a scalp full of dandruff.

Friday 20th July was indeed a day to celebrate as that was the day of my first post-operative shower. Nurse Misaki came to prepare my leg dressings and systematically wrapped the lower tibial area with cling film, finished on each end with five centimetre wide opaque medical tape. After grabbing my towel and shower kit, she held my wheelchair while I somewhat clumsily got up, twisted my body around and eased myself into the chair, making sure my right leg was aligned along the leg extender support. She then pushed me along to the shower rooms which were located directly in front of the large lifts. This was a small area with two washing machines, two driers and a sink in the middle with four shower rooms on the left and one to the right. The first shower room on the left was big enough for a wheelchair. The three other showers were single, narrow cubicles, much like one might have at home. None of these were suitable for me as I was taking up too much space in the wheelchair because of my extended leg. The shower room I would use while in the wheelchair with leg extended would be the one on the right. It was a spacious tiled room about three metres long by two metres wide and had two hair washing sinks at the far end. Nurse Misaki had to help me at this stage to get out of my wheelchair at the drier end of the room to the foam padded shower chair at the wet end of the room, which may sound like an easy task given the short distance of a metre or so but it was quite tricky considering the floor was wet and that my right leg was completely useless as a support. She helped lift my leg onto another shower stool in front of me as it had to be raised at all times. If the leg was down in the normal vertical position, within ten seconds blood would rush to my foot and not be able to return anywhere near as quickly, resulting in pain and discolouration.

As I undressed, I handed over my clothes, underwear and all, to Nurse Misaki so she could place them in the basket at the top of the room behind a shower curtain, another reminder that I'd left my dignity at the hospital entrance and wouldn't be able to pick it up again until the day I was discharged. When she was satisfied that I was in a safe position to shower, she left me to my own devices. When she returned some fifteen minutes later, after I had showered and dried myself, she assisted me in getting dressed and swinging back into my wheelchair. I reveled in the feeling of being clean again.

Shower days were limited and I could only shower on a Tuesday and a Friday morning. In my room, Ryuji San and I used to cheer when shower days came. "Shower Time!" would be known as "Show Time!" from the first time, as Ryuji San misheard the former for the latter. So in addition to the movies we watched everyday, we had "Show Time!" twice a week.

For the first few days, cling film was used to keep both dressings and wounds dry, but after that, Dr. Tsuchiya used special white waterproof plaster dressings, in varying sizes, to dress the incision wounds and a large one with a soft honeycomb backing on it for the long trauma wound. The honeycomb cushioning was designed to give some protection and allow any blood or fluid to be clearly visible. Those dressings remained on my leg for two or three days, and a black permanent marker was used to outline the edge of the blood stain each day, as it slowly soaked across the white sterile surface of the plaster, so it could easily be compared with subsequent stains.

Both dressings and sterile double valve peripheral intravenous catheter needed to be changed every four or five days. On the intravenous kit, the date was marked with a permanent marker pen on the adhesive dressing holding the needle and cannula in place. I dreaded those moments, not because removing the long cannula hurt, I hardly flinched; what ***did*** hurt was the removal of the adhesive patch. As female nurses don't usually sport hairy arms and legs, they thought they were being gentle by peeling off adhesive strips and plaster dressings ***very slowly***, but as any man with hair on his arms knows, peeling slowly hurts even more. I demonstrated one day to the duty nurse, the least painful way to remove an adhesive patch from a man's hairy arm. With her scissors, I first of all made a cut along the length of the needle base and peeled back the tape each side of the cut to free it from the cannula housing. Then I asked her to hold down the whole housing while I counted to three and quickly whipped off the patch, now covered in hairs. In Japanese, she exclaimed *"No, no! I could not do that!"* to which I quickly responded, ***"So you'd rather inflict pain?"***, which brought shrieks of laughter throughout the room.

On the morning of 24th July, Dr. Tsuchiya's immediate boss, Dr. Hyodo, came to see me to ask if I wouldn't mind moving to another room, on the fifth floor. I could hardly refuse, but I wasn't happy with the move at the time. Not only was it so sudden, but I had settled in well in Room 8002 and instead of staring into a sea of conversation killing drapes, in Ryuji San I had someone to talk to at practically any time of the day. One of the ward assistants came to my bed space about thirty minutes later with a small two-tier stainless steel trolley. It was barely big enough for all the stuff I had accumulated while in hospital. She had brought along two clear plastic 100 ltr bags and I threw as much as I could into them after emptying the bedside unit. The unknown was waiting for me three floors down and I had no choice but to pack up and abandon ship.

I had gotten to know all the nurses and ward assistants on A Team, the administration staff in the nurse station and other patients in the ward and it had required a lot of effort on my part. Everyday, I laughed and joked with the nurses, Ryuji San and other patients. Although I was in a hospital ward, I felt quite comfortable. This had become a good place to rest my bones and rehabilitate. So when I reached my new room, 5053, on the fifth floor, I really didn't feel like making much of an effort to communicate as I had done on the eighth floor. Somehow, I had become a stranger again and for a while I still felt attached to my former room on the eighth floor. However, I was going to be here for at least another month so I made an effort to get to know the nurses, administration staff, other patients on the same floor, and of course my new room mates. I still visited the eighth floor from time to time to say hello and wile a bit of time away catching up with all those whose friendship I'd previously acquired.

The layout of the fifth floor was exactly the same as the eighth so navigating my way around was a *'piece of cake'*. The room numbers were of course different but the greatest difference became a great benefit to me; the view out of the window. I had been under the care of A Team of 8F East Nurse Station and enjoyed a reasonably good view extending out towards Yokohama. There were no tall buildings between Motosumiyoshi and the city of Yokohama and therefore the view was exceptionally wide, with the Toyoko and Meguro Lines to the right and Nakahara Heiwa Park to the left.

However, now I had a window seat for a completely different view. I was now under the command of Alpha Team of the West Nurse Station and they afforded me a spectacular view of the skyline of Musashikosugi and what a fabulous skyline it was, not terribly so during the day, but one which came alive at night between the blue-lit strip lighting around the edges of the graduating roof and the array of lights beaming out of a multitude of apartments like the light emitting diodes (L.E.D.) activated on the flight deck of a 777 in cruise, at night. The view was definitely a compensation for having to leave the eighth floor. I enjoyed watching movies almost every night, with the curtains open and that spectacular view as a backdrop.

After unpacking all my gear and setting up my bed space, one of the nurses came in just to chat to me. This time a male nurse named Kazuhiro Satoh. I had previously heard of him through his friend and fellow male nurse on the eighth floor, Male Nurse Naomi Haemoto. Male Nurse Satoh of course, knew that I was coming to his team. I can imagine there would have been a briefing in the nurse station that morning and chatter among the nurses about some tall, Scottish gentleman joining the patient list.

Ryuji San and I would often chat to Male Nurse Haemoto whenever he was on duty. He was a very good communicator and an excellent, professional nurse. He always spared time to talk or answer questions, as did all the nurses.

During my final week before discharge, I had become a little more engaged in conversation with the three older men who were male patients in the same room as mine. Directly across from me was Suzuki San, a man in his late sixties, with very short trimmed hair and very few teeth. He enjoyed chatting and complaining mildly about things, particularly his situation and his rehabilitation requirements. There was something wrong with his left leg but I could not for the life of me figure out what it was. Diagonally across from me was Yamamoto San, a man in his sixties, with fairly kempt hair and a full set of teeth. He had had an operation at the top of his spine and base of his neck and it had left a long very visible scar, but he was a pleasant fellow and also enjoyed chatting. None of them spoke any English so I always had to converse in Japanese. Yamamoto San and Suzuki San often talked together, even after lights were out.

My nearest neighbour, to my right was Nara San who was the oldest, in his late seventies. He was of frail build and always moved around in his wheelchair as he had had his right foot amputated. He had been issued with a prosthetic foot but I never saw him use it. He never really spoke to me until the last couple of days, although I always initiated morning greetings to him to which he would respond. He was hard of hearing too so I needed to talk fairly loudly to him. He never made any effort to engage in conversation with anyone in the room, but he seemed to enjoy drawing attention to himself as he made plenty of noise dropping things like his chopsticks. On one occasion he managed to startle me when he dropped his whole dinner tray. He often pulled the curtains back and forward when he left his bed space and would wander in and out of the room at a very slow pace in his wheelchair, so much so that the tyres would make a slight screeching sound. At night, all three men would raise the noise level by making regurgitating noises whilst clearing their throats, snoring incessantly or demonstrating their fervent passion for breaking wind! I even heard, on more than one occasion, one of the men breaking wind whilst simultaneously snoring. I didn't think that was humanly possible.

One morning when the other two men were out of the room, Nara San drew his wheelchair up towards the window in line with the end of my bed to view out of the window and suddenly started talking to me. I responded of course, but it became mostly a listening exercise for me. I could only catch half of the conversation anyway so correct timing to add to the conversation was proving a challenge. He did though, supported with some clear hand gesture, make a point of complaining about Suzuki San and Yamamoto San chatting all the time, especially at night. I could hardly disagree. To me, that was very amusing in itself because when Nara San was out of the room, Suzuki San would do exactly the same, complaining about Nara San, using similar body language to get his message across. I could hardly disagree.

I got the impression Nara San was a little sad that I was leaving and that was one reason he began to speak more to me. He obviously didn't speak much to the other two. I can't work out why he left it until the last couple of days though when I had been in the room for more than six weeks.

One of Suzuki San's pet complaints was of an elderly woman who was in one of the few single rooms on the other side of the corridor. There was obviously something wrong with her mentally as well, for every morning, afternoon and evening, without fail, she would call out to anyone passing by to summon a nurse as she desperately needed to visit the toilet. I soon learned on reporting to the ward nurse that this constant repetition was a symptom of her dementia and that she didn't really require to use the toilet. When she called out to the nurses every time they passed that she needed the toilet desperately and couldn't wait, they always responded politely with the same phlegmatic response ***"Just a moment please, I'm dealing with another patient right now"***.

She would often catch visitors out, who would then run up to the nurse station only to discover it was a false alarm. Her wolf cries were only exasperating Suzuki San. In the evening, he would slide the room door closed, before a nurse would open it again and ask him not to close the door. His only solution was to switch the bedside television on and don his earphones. A few days before my discharge, the old lady was transferred to another hospital but the silence of her absence soon after was broken by a new voice in the distance, calling out, ***"Who are you? Who are you? Who is there?"***. Suzuki San simply sighed and raised his hands in the air, as if to give in. Of course, these poor women could not help themselves and it was sad to witness their plight. They were entitled to the same medical treatment as every other patient in the hospital but their special needs and constant cries were often very disturbing for other patients who required sleep and rest in order to recover.

The nursing staff had a tough job at times, but even so, every one of the nurses was genuinely pleasant and not one of them ever complained or changed the tone of their voice to demonstrate tiredness, disgust or disapproval, regardless of any apparent annoyance from patients. If there was a hospital paradise, this was surely it.

Chapter Six
Seiken

After returning from the operating theatre, I was administered saline solution for the first twelve hours or so. Around that time, a female medical intern came to my bed with Nurse Asami to insert an intravenous needle and catheter into a vein in my left forearm. I was pretty used to having my veins punctured by ultra sharp double-bevelled needles by this stage so another one to me was just a part of the process of my recovery. It must have been just before lights out, around nine o'clock, as the intern located a nice big juicy vein to puncture. She was very gentle about it, perhaps even a little nervous, seeing as she wasn't yet a certified doctor. She then picked up an alcohol swab from the small blue basket that Nurse Asami had prepared, tore it open and cleaned the target area. Nurse Asami then handed her the needle and after pulling off the sheath, inserted it smoothly into my arm and blood immediately filled the small plastic tubing attached to the needle base, short of the closed plastic valve. With her left thumb, she held the cannula in place and with her right hand, placed a special thin clear plastic adhesive square to hold it permanently and finished off by wrapping a circular expandable bandage cover over it to keep the two plastic pipes and blue one-way end valves in place.

Some twenty minutes later, Nurse Asami placed an intravenous bag on a hook at the top of the mobile I.V. pole and connected the plastic tubing from the bag to one of the blue valves connected to the needle base. She then unwrapped a sterile, disposable syringe filled with saline solution and connected that to the other, venting valve, slowly pumping the saline into the tube to clear any air between the needle and the intravenous agent, ensuring flow of the agent into my vein. I could feel the rush of saline punch up through my vein as it was slightly cooler than my body temperature. Then, synchronising with her watch, she checked the rate of flow as it entered my bloodstream. That agent was the antibiotic, cefazolin (*Rasenazolin*®). If I forgot all other antibiotics I ever had in my life, this is one antibiotic I will never forget. Cefazolin will be forever etched on my mind.

I noticed the initial symptoms within the first twenty four hours when Nurse Misaki came to take my daily blood pressure and temperature readings. I felt excessively warm but the air conditioning was on in the room so it couldn't have been as warm as it appeared to me at the time. My blood pressure was normal but my body temperature was 37.8, a little high. I was able to take my own temperature anytime as the thermometer was kept in a little pocket attached to the bed railing. As the day wore on, I monitored my temperature. It was rising. By evening, my temperature had risen to 38 degrees and I was becoming quite uncomfortable. I requested two 'kori makuras' (ice pillows), together with the painkillers I had been taking and some medicine to help me sleep.

I was also given 400mg of Ibuprofen to alleviate my post-surgery pain. Ibuprofen is a non-steroidal anti-inflammatory drug (NSAID) and works by reducing hormones that cause inflammation and pain in the body.[19] The sleeping medicine I was given was *Brotizolam®*, 0.25mg, which is a sedative-hypnotic thienodiazepine drug. It possesses anxiolytic, anticonvulsant, hypnotic, sedative and skeletal muscle relaxant properties. Brotizolam is an extremely potent drug and it is rapidly eliminated with an average half-life of 4.4 hours (range 3.6 – 7.9 hours), so given the fact that I had taken it at 8:00pm as I would be awoken at 06:30am as usual, I expected it to help me fall asleep around 10:00pm. Here I was using it in Japan, but

---

[19] *http://www.drugs.com/ibuprofen.html*

brotizolam is not approved for sale in the UK, United States or Canada.[20]

I had some trouble getting to sleep that night, even with the sleeping medication but when I awoke in the morning, my temperature had not changed. By late afternoon my temperature had actually continued to rise and now with the onset of fever it was 39.8. The nurses monitored me closely.

My temperature at this stage was high and constant but I was shivering uncontrollably in bed and experiencing phases of feeling cold and feeling hot. I felt dreadful as I lay in bed during the day, shivering under the double bedsheets, but the worst was yet to come.

As afternoon turned to evening, my skin became incredibly itchy and I had to try really hard to resist scratching for I knew my skin could be left open to infection or at the very least be left with ugly scars. My whole body was hot and itchy and my skin was turning red. Worse still, my hands and arms were suffering from a severe case of edematous swelling, meaning that an excessive accumulation of serous fluid was building up in the tissue spaces below my skin. I not only needed brotizolam to sleep, more urgently I needed ice. The nurse gave me four ice pillows and filled up my own ice pack. The immediate cooling

---

[20] *http://www.drugbank.ca/drugs/DB09017*

sensation was such a relief, but I was still in a fever, my skin was all red and my hands and arms were swollen. I had no idea what was happening to me but I knew it wasn't normal. I guess the only fortunate thing to say about the whole situation was that I was at least in a hospital.

In the morning, my intermittent fever was still with me and my temperature was still in the 39 degree range. The swelling was much worse and had now spread to my face; my head displayed edematous swelling, my eyes were puffed up and my ears were red. My whole face felt like it had been used as a hot punchbag and my back was incredibly warm and uncomfortable. At that point I assumed it was due to the heat from my body warming up the thin, stiff foam mattress on which I was lying, but in addition to it being very itchy, I could feel a distinct lump there. In fact, I could feel a large area of lumps. I was unable to inspect the area myself so I asked one of the nurses to check it for me. She was surprised at what she saw. I handed her my iPhone and asked her to take a photograph. I too was shocked to see my back. It was covered in large red lumps and there were rash spots all over my skin, particularly concentrated on my lower spinal area, but what was more worrying was the fact that it was spreading to my arms and face. I looked and felt absolutely awful.

A little time later, a female dermatologist, Dr. Kitajima, came to see me and inspect my skin condition. She suspected I had either hives or urticaria but couldn't immediately explain what was causing them. She said she would prescribe medication to relieve the itching in the meantime and would visit me the following day to see if there was any change.

About an hour after her visit, one of the pharmacists arrived with the medicines Dr. Kitajima had prescribed. Three of the items were ointments, one of which was a white ointment called Antebate Ointment 0.05%, a 5g steroid preparation containing *betamethasone butyrate propionate* (steroid that reduces inflammation throughout the body), which suppresses skin inflammation to improve symptoms such as redness, swelling and itchiness. The second ointment was *Rinderon®-V* cream, containing 0.6mg of *Betamethasone Valerate* (a synthetic adrenocortico-steroid). Rinderon-V is a steroid drug used for the relief of inflammatory and pruritic (itchy) manifestations of corticosteroid-responsive dermatoses (non-inflammatory skin disorder) and itches that may occur with certain skin problems and allergies. It is also used to aid fluid retention in head injuries, to control asthma and may also be used to prevent organ transplant rejection after a transplant.[21] The third ointment,

[21] *http://www.igenericdrugs.com/?s=rinderon-v*

Locoid® contained the topical corticosteroid hydrocortisone butyrate (steroid hormone produced by the adrenal cortex and used medicinally to treat inflammation resulting from eczema and rheumatism), a non-fluorinated hydrocortisone ester and each gram of this ointment contained 1 mg of hydrocortisone butyrate in a base of mineral oil and polyethylene.[22]

I smeared these three ointments all over my body each morning, over the next few days. In addition to the ointments, I was given 2.5mg rebamipide and 5mg of olopatadine hydrochloride, two antihistamines. Apart from suppressing the itchiness somewhat, these drugs didn't reduce the redness or alleviate the rash or swelling.

Dr. Kitajima visited me again with another doctor whose department was clearly stitched on his white coat. It boldly read ***'Department of Infectious Diseases'***. Not a comforting thought at the time. His brief, I suspected, was to inspect my condition with the view of detecting any recognisable symptoms of disease, but the only thing he made disappear very quickly were the three visitors who had come to see me. Dr. Kitajima then asked me if I would be willing to be subjected to a subcutaneous tissue biopsy. In my current state, I thought it was a wise idea, so I agreed to have this done. This procedure would be carried out

---

[22] *http://www.rxlist.com/locoid-drug.htm*

the following morning. Believing it would help to discover what was wrong with me, I didn't really mind and was quite eager to have it done.

After Dr. Kitajima *et al* had left, I carried out some research on the subject. There are several types of skin biopsy methods conducted, according to the suspected diagnosis of the skin lesion. I had agreed to an incisional biopsy. This needs to be performed at the darkest area of pigmentation and the thickest tangible area of the lesion. After the tissue surrounding the lesion is anaesthetised, a scalpel would then be used to make parallel elliptical-shaped incisions through the central part of the lesion, extending at each end into normal tissue. The central part of the lesion would then be removed, thus preserving the histological architecture of the tissue's cells and providing a cross-sectional wedge of tissue for histopathologic analysis (microscopic examination of tissue) by a dermatopathologist. The primary advantage of an incisional biopsy over other methods is that hemostasis can be done more easily due to better visualization.

Next morning, I was taken down to the second floor and to Dr. Kitajima's examination room. Once on the table, with my T-shirt removed, Dr. Kitajima asked if it was okay to take some pictures. I agreed, wondering if I might end up in some medical journal that was reporting a new virus in town. So she grabbed the Nikon D800 DSLR camera with lens ring flash attached which was sitting on the worktop behind her and started taking photos of my back and sides. I felt like a model for a freak magazine.

Just as she had finished the photography project, her boss entered and introduced himself in English. He had also brought an old style analogue tape recorder with him and plugged it into the wall nearby. I assumed he was going to record some dialogue while I was being incised, but instead, he pressed the play button and *'Let it Go!'*, the title song from the movie 'Frozen' started playing. I was almost speechless but it was nice to listen to it, albeit the Japanese version, looping over and over again. It was very thoughtful of him to try to make me feel relaxed, although I was already as relaxed as I could be given the feverish condition I was in.

With the scene set, Dr. Kitajima started to prepare my skin by swabbing with an antiseptic agent, followed by an injection of a local anaesthetic, epinephrine, around the target area, which was halfway down my side. Her assistant then placed a blue fenestrated surgical drape over my side. I was a little disappointed that I couldn't actually see the surgical procedure, as I wanted to video it with my iPhone. In hindsight, I should have stipulated that as a criteria for agreeing to the biopsy.

Although I couldn't feel the pain, I could feel the trail of the scalpel as she made an elliptical cut through my entire dermis down to the subcutaneous fat. Given the numerous white towels that were used during the procedure, I could tell that the incision was releasing a fair amount of blood and that was slowing down the suture stage. After the incision was fully sutured with nylon sutures, she placed a gauze dressing over the area, held in place with surgical tape. The sample was then prepared by being placed in a fixative which stabilized the tissue, to prevent autolysis. This process of fixation terminates any ongoing biochemical reactions and increases the stability of the treated tissues and the sample is subsequently sent to the pathology laboratory for microscopic and culture analysis, the results of which were expected to take around ten days.

Dr. Kitajima visited me over the next few days to change the dressing and make sure the wound was healing and of course to eventually remove the nylon sutures one week later. In the meantime, I still had a fever and my temperature was not coming down.

When Dr. Kitajima visited my bed again, we both got a bit of a shock in a different sense of the word. I had set the adjustable bed so I was slightly upright and was resting my eyes, relaxing to the peaceful sound of ***birdsongradio.com*** when she approached my bed.

Obviously with my eyes closed, I couldn't see her approach but my sixth sense told me there was someone in front of me. She was just leaning over me to tap me gently on the shoulder to wake me up when I simultaneously opened my eyes, and as I had been daydreaming, the sudden presence of her face right above me didn't register immediately as a human being and I barked out in fright which made her jump back a few feet. We both laughed profusely, as did the nurse who was there, together with my room mates, fellow patients, Ryuji and Kota.

Chapter Seven
Prothrombinase

I didn't realise it was possible to become so busy as an in-patient in hospital. A week after my biopsy, on Friday 27th June, Dr. Hyodo came in to see me and let me know that the problem I was having was most likely not a virus or disease but an allergic reaction to the antibiotic I was on. I did wonder at the time why it had taken so long to reach that conclusion so following my discharge from hospital I decided to do some research to see how this apparent delay in the medical team's diagnosis had come about. In the process of my research I found it was not difficult to identify the possibility of an allergic reaction, for reasons I will explain shortly. He said that it was not a good idea though to simply stop the intravenous infusion I was being administered as its purpose was to fight any infection at the trauma site so instead, he arranged for my initial antibiotic to be changed to another.

Since I first discovered I had an allergy to penicillin, I had believed it to be the *only* medicine to which I was allergic and so informed the hospital accordingly to ensure they did not administer as part of my treatment, any drug which contained penicillin or penicillin derivatives.

The initial antibiotic that was causing all the problems was cefazolin sodium. Cefazolin is a first generation cephalosporin antibiotic that works by fighting serious bacteria in the body, but as I later discovered in my research, cefazolin belongs to a group of antibiotics called cephalosporins that work by inhibiting cell wall synthesis of the bacteria which they achieve by binding to penicillin-binding proteins (PBSs). These groups of antibiotics are known as bactericidal, meaning that they kill the targeted bacteria, as opposed to inhibiting reproduction as bacteriostatic antibiotics do. Cefazolin attains high serum levels and is excreted quickly via the urine.[23]

From my research findings, it seemed obvious the conclusion would have been not to administer cefazolin in the first place. However, on further examination of the findings it became clear that cefazolin *was* in fact the most obvious choice due to it being one of the most widely studied antibiotics with proven efficacy and also effective against bone infections. I was intrigued to learn that most cross reactivity between penicillins and cephalosporins

---

[23] *http://www.drugbank.ca/drugs/DB01327*

stems from whether their R1 side chains are structurally similar. Cross reactivity between penicillins and most second- and all third- and fourth-generation cephalosporins is negligible. The overall cross reactivity between penicillins and cephalosporins in individuals who report a penicillin allergy is approximately 1% and, in those with a confirmed penicillin allergy, 2.55%. The University of Maryland, School of Medicine concluded in a 2012 clinical review, that although a myth persisted that approximately 10% of patients with a history of penicillin allergy will have an allergic reaction if given a cephalosporin, the overall cross-reactivity rate was approximately 1% when using first-generation cephalosporins or cephalosporins with similar R1 side chains. For penicillin-allergic patients like myself, the use of third- or fourth-generation cephalosporins or cephalosporins with dissimilar side chains than the offending penicillin would probably have carried a negligible risk of cross allergy.[24] However, I did not know the actual side chain of my offending penicillin at the time and so was unable to provide this information to the hospital. Had I known this information, the hospital may have been able to safely administer a cephalosporin with a side chain that is structurally dissimilar to that of the penicillin I am allergic to, whilst I would receive the most

[24] *The Journal of Emergency Medicine, Volume 42, Issue 5, May 2012, pages 612-620*

appropriate antibiotic to fight the infection in my leg. Based on my own research, if I were to make a clinical elimination of penicillin strains, I would deduce that I have a particular allergy to the Cupriavidus Taiwanensis R1 strain (LMG 19424).

I was immediately disconnected from the 250mg per six hour period of cefazolin I had been receiving. An alternative antibiotic was being prepared in the pharmacy which I would receive shortly. A little later that afternoon, I was requested to visit Radiology to undergo a CT scan. None of my doctors were around so I was unable to confirm the reason for the CT scan until I reached Radiology when the radiologist who greeted me said that I had a suspected *embolism*.

That was not something I expected to hear. An embolism in my case meant the lodging of an embolis, in the form of a *blood clot*, in my bloodstream. That was dangerous and a serious condition as it could have caused vascular occlusion in a blood vessel which may in turn have affected a part of my body distanced from the actual site of the embolism, like my heart or lungs.

In my wheelchair and with fever still hanging over me, I was wheeled into the CT room and up to the motorised bed of the Toshiba Aquilion 64 CT scanner with contrast injector system where I removed my slippers and moved onto the table with my feet at the entrance to the CT scanning gantry. As I lay there on the narrow table, I began to shiver uncontrollably again and started to feel very cold. CT rooms are kept at a cooler temperature than most other areas of a hospital and my body was becoming sensitive to this. The room has to be kept between 18°C (64°F) and 24°C (75°F) as the CT machine generates a lot of heat, which can damage it. In this state, the technician was unable to conduct an accurate scan so long as I was shaking so he draped a couple of large bed terry towels over me and that did the trick after a couple of minutes. I wished I had been in a better condition as I was very interested in the procedure and would have asked questions to demonstrate my interest but I just wanted to get the scanning procedure over with quickly and get back upstairs to bed. I do recall though, once I had stabilised my shaking, that I had watched the technician prepare the machine by inserting a very large clear plastic syringe, containing a contrasting agent into the arm of the Covidien Optistar Elite Contrast Injector arm and connected that to the intravenous administration catheter that was already in my forearm. As the CT table was moved through the scanning ring on its initial phase, leaving my head just in front of the 720mm diameter scanning gantry, I found it increasingly difficult to stay perfectly still. I was relieved when the X-ray induction motors whirred down for a couple of minutes while the technician attended to some settings. I really began to feel like I was in a '**Terminator**' movie as the machine started up again and a large mechanical arm moved out towards me. When the arm stopped, the X-ray induction motors started up again and that familiar spinning noise returned. This time, the table moved further into the scanning gantry and stopped. After a pause of a few seconds, a piston on the arm pushed down on the top of the syringe and promptly administered 370mg of *Oypalomin®*, the radiographic contrast medium, through the flexible intravenous cannula and into my veins. I can only describe this sensation as similar to having a reasonably hot cup of tea flow through your veins from head to foot. This was the weird experience I had been told to expect, as the contrast agent flowed very quickly through my body. At the same time, as if following the flow of the contrast agent as it past down through my body, the table brought my whole body back up through scanning gantry until my feet were clear. Mission complete. At 6:34pm on Friday 27th June 2014, I had been tomographically scanned.

After leaving Radiology, I was wheeled back to my room where I just crawled back onto the bed, pulled the two bed sheets over me and closed my eyes. I was barely in a twenty minute sleep when I was awoken by a Japanese friend whom I had been expecting. At that point a doctor appeared and my visitor politely left to allow the doctor to attend to me in private. The doctor arrived carrying a basket containing at least one hypodermic syringe and several glass tubes to collect blood samples.

I'd rather any doctor or nurse drawing blood from me would refrain from saying ***"this might hurt a bit"*** as my mind quickly shifts to the anticipation and inevitability of pain. He said I was suspected of having ***venous thromboembolism (VTE)*** and he needed to draw a sample of blood from three different locations. Firstly from my forearm, which thankfully was painless, probably as I had become accustomed to this frequent procedure. Then he drew a sample from my foot, which did hurt a little, and finally, he inserted a syringe right down into my femoral artery, close to the inguinal ligament in my lower groin area and that ***really*** hurt; so much so, my eyes widened and my back arched as expelled air hissed from my gritted teeth. I did not want to go through that ***ever*** again.

Less than an hour later, the duty night nurse came in with a small square, cream coloured machine with a digital screen, attached to a mobile stainless steel I.V. pole and a 500ml bag of low molecular weight heparin (LMWH). LMWH was used as it has a lower risk of heparin-induced thrombocytopenia compared with unfractionated heparin. The device delivering the heparin was the Terumo TE-112, a 100v controlled dosage infusion pump. Its purpose was to control the amount of anticoagulant being administered through the sterile intravenous cannula in the vein in my arm, to 10ml per hour. I had no idea at the time though that I would be connected to this machine practically twenty four hours a day for the next two weeks.

Heparin is a naturally occurring polysaccharide that inhibits blood coagulation, the process that leads to thrombosis.[25] Discovered in 1916, heparin is one of the most effective and widely used drugs of this century. It is prepared by extraction from the tissue of slaughter house animals (i.e., porcine intestine, bovine lung).[26] The use of heparin and LMWHs can sometimes result in a decrease in platelet count, known as Heparin Induced Thrombocytopenia.[27]

In addition to the heparin, I was administered a new antibiotic, clindamycin. Clindamycin is useful for the treatment of a number of infections, belonging to the lincosamide class, but is usually used to treat infections with anaerobic bacteria.[28]

---

[25] *New England Journal of Medicine 1997 Sep 4;337(10):688-98*

[26] *Department of Medicinal and Natural Products Chemistry, University of Iowa, "Production and Chemical Processing of Low Molecular Weight Heparins"*

[27] *Prevention and treatment of venous thromboembolism. International Consensus Statement (Guidelines according to scientific evidence). Int Angiol 2006; 25:101-161*

[28] *"Clinical practice. Skin and soft-tissue infections caused by methicillin-resistant Staphylococcus aureus". New England Medical Journal, 2007 357 (4): 380–90*

Furthermore, as a precaution, I also underwent a continuous saline infusion to flush my kidneys, with a saline solution connected to an intravenous bag hanging from an I.V. pole on the other side of the bed, which in turn was connected to a sterile intravenous administration kit and cannula in my right arm. For the first forty eight hours, I was pretty much bed bound and every time I needed to go to the toilet, I had to make a nurse call. The duty nurse would respond and remove the saline bag from its stand and hang it to the heparin and clindamycin stand, then unplug the infusion pump, which would then obtain its power from a back up battery, while I moved into my wheelchair. The nurse would then wheel me to the toilet, while I steered the I.V. pole with my hands. With the 'Call of Nature' finished, I would wash my hands and press the nurse call button and wait to be wheeled back to my bed to be re-connected to the relevant monitors and IV links.

There was one other piece of equipment with which I had been issued during the heparin administration period and that was a lightweight, hand-held Electro Cardiograph (ECG) device. Connected to that was an 80cm long 3-lead electrode cable leading to three 35mm foam taped, solid gel vitrode electrodes on the ends so as to record the transthoracic interpretation of the electrical activity of my heart in addition to an *SpO2* (estimation of the oxygen saturation level and measurement of the percentage of hemoglobin binding sites in the bloodstream occupied by oxygen) with a finger sensor. This device could wirelessly transmit live-monitoring data directly to a central monitor in the nurse station, thus generating automatic data integration into the hospital electronic charting system. It would also emit an audio alarm in the nurse station if there was any abnormal electrical activity.

All together, it was a tough weekend. When Monday morning arrived and Dr. Tsuchiya presented the results of my CT scan, I was shocked to discover I had been diagnosed with *distal Deep Vein Thrombosis (DVT), a manifestation of Venous Thromboembolism (VTE).* Venous thromboembolism is a condition that includes both deep vein thrombosis and pulmonary embolism (PE). The CT scan had identified three small but distinctive embolisms about three or four centimetres out from my tibia and towards the proximal end which were clearly shown on several of the CT tomograms. This was just more bad news on top of that I was already suffering. I began to wonder what would be next.

My distal thrombosis was caused by transient risk factors, i.e., a combination of post-surgery fat embolism due to the mobilisation of fluid fat as a result of the trauma to my tibia, fibula and soft tissue, as well as my immobilisation at the time. Fat emboli occur in almost 90% of all patients with severe injuries to bones, although only 10% of these are symptomatic.[29] However, it was critical that therapy began without delay since pulmonary embolism, a potentially life threatening condition, will occur in approximately 50% of untreated individuals.

Although my fever had fallen by that time, my body was still suffering from edematous swelling and covered in rash, but I was a little more comfortable and continued my evening's entertainment provided by my Apple environment. The following evening turned out to be quite amusing for the duty nurse and myself. At the time, as it was lights off, being after 9:00pm, I was watching the sci-fi thriller movie 'Skyline' with earphones plugged in. Suddenly a nurse came to my bedside and asked if I was alright as an alarm had gone off in the nurse station, indicating that I was experiencing abnormal heart activity. When she discovered I was watching a horror movie, we both laughed.

I was also issued with a pair of L-sized Ansilk-Pro J, a Japanese brand of anti-embolism calf compression stockings. These were used to support venous blood return and reduce the possibility of

---

[29] *SURGERY TODAY Volume 37, Number 1, 5–8*

further embolism. These white stockings have a three dimensional structure, fitting to the shape of the leg and the compression design provides a 38% increase in blood pressure, so they constantly give adequate pressure while in the horizontal position; 18mmHg around the ankle, moving through 14mmHg at the calf and 8mmHg just below the knee, though I found them too warm to be comfortable.

Several days had gone by and I still had the rash and edematous swelling, so once again the antibiotic was changed, this time to Vancomycin. Vancomycin is of the glycopeptide antibiotic class and is effective mostly against gram-positive bacteria. The drug was first isolated in 1953 at the U.S. pharmaceutical company, Eli Lilly, from a soil sample collected from the interior jungles of Borneo by a missionary. It is a naturally occurring antibiotic made by the soil bacterium Actinobacteria, species Amycolatopsis Orientalis (genus of gram-positive, filamentous bacteria). It is a complex chemical compound and an example of a comparatively rare halo-organic natural compound, containing two covalently bonded chlorine atoms. The compound was industrially produced by fermentation and given the generic name vancomycin, derived from the term "vanquish". The original indication for vancomycin was for the treatment of penicillin-resistant Staphylococcus aureus, a use kept alive for many years because that compound had to be given intravenously and thus provided bacteria fewer opportunities to evolve resistance, and because organisms were relatively slow to evolve or adapt to it, even in experiments.[30] Vancomycin is recommended to be administered in a dilute solution slowly, over at least 60 minutes (maximum rate of 10 mg/minute for doses >500 mg) due to the high incidence of pain and thrombophlebitis.[31]

However, even vancomycin was not helping to alleviate my symptoms and once again, my antibiotic was changed, this time to Daptomycin. Unlike vancomycin, daptomycin is a cyclic lipopeptide antibiotic that has a unique mechanism of action. It binds to the bacterial cell membranes, causing rapid depolarization of the membrane due to K efflux and associated disruption of Deoxyribonucleic acid (DNA), Ribonucleic acid (RNA), and protein synthesis; the result is rapid bacterial death. Interestingly and perhaps ironically, daptomycin is used mainly for infections caused by vancomycin.[32]

Finally, after administration of the fourth antibiotic, my symptoms started to improve. The

---

[30] *http://www.idsociety.org/uploadedfiles/idsa/guidelines-patient_care/pdf_library/mrsa.pdf*

[31] *"Red man syndrome", Critical care (London, England) 2003, 7 (2): 119–20*

[32] *http://www.merckmanuals.com/professional/infectious_diseases/bacteria_and_antibacterial_drugs/daptomycin.html*

swelling in my face, arms and torso reduced and my skin returned to normal. The itchiness was no more and the rash began to disappear. I had been so pre-occupied with everything that was happening to my body during this difficult period of cross reaction with the cefazolin, that I almost forgot the very reason I was in hospital in the first place. My fractured leg had been put on the shelf.

The intravenous daptomycin course lasted four days and during that period I continued to be connected to the infusion pump feeding me heparin. It proved practically impossible to leave the room other than to visit the toilet over the course of the next two weeks. The heparin infusion was just the initial therapy of anticoagulation though. Normally I should have been administered intravenous heparin for only a few days and then transitioned slowly onto an oral anticoagulant, in this case, Warfarin. Warfarin cannot be administered as a single agent during initiation and has to be given alongside another anti-coagulant, namely, the heparin, and for a minimum period of four to five days.

Before I could be prescribed warfarin and taken off the heparin, my blood clotting time had to be analysed and until it reached a certain score on a blood test, I had to remain on heparin and consequently tied to the infusion pump.

Over the period 27th June to 14th July, I had blood samples drawn a further nine times. The purpose was to subject the samples to a prothrombin (PT) test, or International Normalized Ratio (INR), the latter which is used to standardise the results as different labs use different tests.

Prothrombin itself is a glycoprotein produced by the liver and is an essential component of the blood clotting mechanism occurring in blood plasma.

Prothrombin time was discovered by Dr. Armand Quick and colleagues in 1935.[33] The INR was invented in the early 1980s by Tom Kirkwood working at the UK National Institute for Biological Standards and Control to provide a consistent way of expressing the prothrombin time ratio, which had previously suffered from a large degree of variation between centres using different reagents. The INR became widely accepted worldwide, especially after endorsement by the World Health Organisation.[34]

The PT-INR test the hospital laboratory would perform would be a measure of the extrinsic pathway of my blood coagulation, in other words, how long it took for my blood to coagulate. The necessary

---

[33] *"A study of the coagulation defect in hemophilia and in jaundice". Am J Med Sci 1935, 190 (4): 501*

[34] *"Expert Committee on Biological Standardization. Requirements for thromboplastins and plasma used to control oral anticoagulant therapy". World Health Organ Tech Rep Ser. 1983, pp. 81–105*

therapeutic range for the PT-INR test results needed to be between 2.0 and 3.0 for two consecutive days.

While I was waiting for the results of these PT-INR tests, I continued my research on anticoagulation and the drug I was so desperately waiting to be administered. I discovered that warfarin is the main oral anticoagulant used in the U.K.[35] and the most widely prescribed oral anticoagulant drug in North America and I was informed it was hospital policy to use warfarin here in Japan.

Warfarin is a synthetic derivative of dicoumarol (potent anticoagulant that acts by inhibiting the synthesis of vitamin K-dependent clotting factors in the liver), a 4-hydroxycoumarin-derived mycotoxin anticoagulant originally discovered in spoiled sweet clover-based animal feeds. The name 'warfarin' stems from its discovery at the University of Wisconsin, incorporating the acronym for the organization that funded the key research, "WARF" for the Wisconsin Alumni Research Foundation and the ending "-arin", indicating its link with coumarin (a natural fragrant organic substance found in many plants). It is used to decrease the tendency for thrombosis and can help prevent

[35] *http://www.nhs.uk/conditions/anticoagulants-warfarin-/Pages/Introduction.aspx*

formation of future blood clots and help reduce the risk of embolism.[36]

It was initially introduced in 1948 as a pesticide against rats and mice, and is still used for this purpose. In 1954, it was approved for use as a medication, and has remained popular ever since.[37] Despite its effectiveness, treatment with warfarin has several shortcomings. Many commonly used medications interact with warfarin, as do some foods, particularly grapefruit, natto and leaf vegetable foods or "greens," since these typically contain large amounts of vitamin K, and its activity has to be monitored by INR blood testing to ensure an adequate yet safe dose is taken.[38]

As I mentioned, it was hospital policy to prescribe warfarin as the drug choice for oral anticoagulation but I found a newer, orally active anticoagulant drug called Rivaroxiban, during the course of my research, which demonstrated similar efficacy to warfarin. Unlike the K-antagonist warfarin, rivaroxiban is an Xa inhibitor which meant that it could be given as a fixed dose oral agent, thus eliminating the need for further laboratory monitoring

---

[36] *The American Society of Health-System Pharmacists. Retrieved 3 April 2011*

[37] *"Systematic overview of warfarin and its drug and food interactions". Arch. Intern. Med. 2005, 165 (10): 1095–106*

[38] *"Pharmacology and management of the vitamin K antagonists: American College of Chest Physicians evidence-based clinical practice guidelines (8th Edition)". Chest 2008, 133 (6 Suppl): 160S–198*

and hospital visits to have blood samples taken. Furthermore, rivaroxiban was proven to be superior for the prevention of recurrent DVT and a prolonged period of bridging therapy would not be necessary which would mean a shorter transition from the heparin course.[39]

There were of course some disadvantages to this drug. According to one of the hospital pharmacists who came to see me, the cost of a daily dose of my 4.5mg of warfarin was ¥43 (approx. $0.40), whereas the 20mg of rivaroxiban I'd need for a daily dose[40] was ¥766[41] (approx. $7.11), almost eighteen times more expensive. Additionally, being a new drug, it did not have a readily available antidote for bleeding events that might occur and there was also a lack of clarification on long term safety and drug-drug interactions. In the end, it wasn't possible to have rivaroxiban anyway, for although the pharmacy had stock of the drug, and it has been approved in over one hundred countries worldwide as a treatment for DVT, it had not yet been approved by the Japanese Ministry of Health, Labor and Welfare (JMHLW) for use as an

---

[39] *http://www.uptodate.com/contents/treatment-of-lower-extremity-deep-vein-thrombosis?source=search_result&search=Treatment+of+lower+extremity+deep+vein+thrombosis&selectedTitle=1%7E150*

[40] *http://www.rxfiles.ca/rxfiles/uploads/documents/ROCKET-AF-Rivaroxaban.pdf*

[41] *http://www.qlife.jp/meds/rx33920.html*

oral anticoagulant. In 2012, the pharmaceutical company Bayer Healthcare obtained approval to market the drug, under the brand name *Xarelto®*, for the prevention of stroke and systemic embolism in patients with non-valvular atrial fibrillation,[42] but although in May 2014, it submitted an application to JMHLW for approval to market the drug as an anticoagulant for DVT and PE[43], approval was still pending during my time in hospital.

I had no choice but to accept the warfarin. My initial dose was 10mg, then adjusted to 8mg after two days then further adjusted to 5mg. After subsequent PT-INR testing, the dosage dropped to 4mg and then stabilised at 4.5mg. At this stage, I needed to give blood to have the samples INR-monitored every three to four weeks for a minimum period of two months. Interestingly, there are few studies that offer guidance on the appropriate length of treatment of patients with provoked symptomatic distal thrombosis.[44]

---

42 *http://press.healthcare.bayer.com/en/press/news-details-page.php/14463/2012-0019*

43 *http://www.pharmaceuticalonline.com/doc/bayer-files-xarelto-application-to-treat-dvt-pe-in-japan-0001*

44 *http://www.uptodate.com/contents/treatment-of-lower-extremity-deep-vein-thrombosis?source=search_result&search=Treatment+of+lower+extremity+deep+vein+thrombosis&selectedTitle=1%7E150*

Chapter Eight
Rehabiri

A host of reactions are going on inside muscle, bone, tissue and flesh after trauma. At cellular level, pathologic changes include the shrinkage of muscle fibres, the loss of nuclei from multi-nucleated muscle cells, and a series of apoptosis events, the process of programmed cell death.

To put the repair process into a biological perspective, immediately after my initial trauma and deterioration of muscle tone, the tissue at the injury site was forming *hematoma* (localized swelling that is filled with blood caused by a break in the wall of a blood vessel), with obvious inflammation, and at the same time, the myofibres in my lower leg muscles were rupturing and my bone cells were *necrotising* (causing the death of tissues). During this first phase, the inflammatory cells were able to freely invade the injury site because the blood vessels were torn although this is an essential component of the healing process.

The most abundant inflammatory cells are the *polymorphonuclear leukocytes* (a type of white blood cell that helps the body fight off infection). These were replaced by *monocytes* (large white blood cells with a simple oval nucleus and clear, grayish fluid that fills the cell), a few hours after my injury. These cells eventually transformed into *macrophages* (large cells found in stationary form in the tissues or as a mobile white blood cell, especially at sites of infection). Macrophages assumed two specific functions. Firstly, they removed the necrotic myofibres by a process known as *phagocytosis* (wherein certain living cells called phagocytes ingest or engulf other cells or particles). Secondly, they produced, together with *fibroblasts* (a type of cell that is responsible for making the extracellular matrix and collagen), chemotactic signals such as growth factors, *cytokines* (small proteins released by cells that have a specific effect on the interactions between cells, on communication between cells or on the behaviour of cells), and *chemokines* (a family of small cytokines, or signaling proteins secreted by cells). The *extracellular matrix* (ECM) (a collection of extracellular molecules secreted by cells that provide structural and biochemical support to the surrounding cells) also contained growth factors that became active when the tissue in my lower leg was damaged. Some of these growth factors were able to activate *myogenic precursors* (substances originating in muscle tissue from which another is formed, especially by metabolic reaction), called satellite cells.[45]

The next phase, referred to as the repair phase, consisted of two concomitant processes. The first was the regeneration of the disrupted myofibres. Regeneration can occur because there is still a pool of undifferentiated reserve cells, also called myogenic precursors or satellite cells under the *basal lamina* (thin, planar assembly of extracellular matrix proteins which supports all epithelia, muscle cells, and nerve cells outside the central nervous system) of the myofibre. The satellite cells experienced a process of proliferation, i.e., the reproduction or multiplication of similar forms and eventually differentiated into *myoblasts* (embryonic cells that become cells of muscle fibres). The second process of the repair phase is the formation of a connective tissue scar by *fibrin* (protein that is formed during normal blood clotting and that is the essence of the clot) and *fibronectin* (fibrous protein that binds to collagen, fibrin, and other proteins and also to the cell membranes, functioning as an anchor and connector), derived from blood of the hematoma that was formed immediately after my injury. The scar tissue gave my muscles strength to withstand

45 *"Muscle injuries: biology and treatment," American Journal of Sports Medicine, vol. 33, no. 5, pp. 745–764, 2005*

contractions. However, if there had been excessive proliferation of these fibroblasts, dense scar tissue would have formed within the injured muscle. This would not only interfere with the repair process but would also interrupt the muscle regenerative process and contribute to incomplete functional recovery of the injured muscle during the third phase, referred to as the remodeling phase. In this last phase, the newly formed myofibres mature. At the same time, the scar tissue is reorganized and it contracts.[46]

Over the next three to four weeks, it was confirmed by my surgeon's examination of my x-ray results that the regenerative process had begun to develop with the growth of *fibrocartilaginous callus* (temporary formation of cells which formed at the area of the bone fracture as the bone attempted to heal itself) through the process of capillary growth in the hematoma, the invasion and cleaning up of debris in the injury site by *phagocytic cells* (cells, such as white blood cells, that engulf and absorb waste material, harmful micro-organisms, or other foreign bodies in the bloodstream and tissues), and the migration into the site by *fibroblasts* (cells that are responsible for making the extracellular matrix and collagen) and *osteoblasts* (cells that secrete the matrix for bone

---

[46] *"Differentiation repertoire of fibroblastic cells: expression of cytoskeletal proteins as marker of phenotypic modulations," Laboratory Investigation, vol. 63, no. 2, pp. 144–161, 1990*

formation) marking the reconstruction of my tibia. Around the fourth week, my lateral X-ray images showed evidence of bone callus formation. This process is enacted by the multiplying of osteoblasts and *osteocytes* (bone cells, formed when an osteoblast becomes embedded in the matrix it has secreted), resulting in fibrocartilaginous callus turning into bony callus. The process of tissue regeneration and scar formation is orderly but complex.

However, complete recovery from my injury was compromised due to the development of *fibrosis* (formation of excess fibrous connective tissue in the reparative process) in the second week after the injury. The formed scar tissue is always mechanically inferior and therefore much less able to perform the functions of a normal muscle fibre. It is also more susceptible to re-injury.[47] To minimize the disability and enhance full functional recovery after my surgery, treatment included limiting the bleeding with compression, elevation, and local cooling, and of course physical therapy[48]

Continued inactivity can lead to *atrophy* (shrinking or wasting of a body part as a result of lack

---

[47] *"Growth factors improve muscle healing in vivo," Journal of Bone and Joint Surgery B, vol. 82, no. 1, pp. 131–137, 2000*

[48] *"Muscle injuries: biology and treatment," American Journal of Sports Medicine, vol. 33, no. 5, pp. 745–764, 2005*

of use) of the healthy muscles whereas early mobilization accelerates capillary ingrowth and promotes the regeneration of muscle fibres. However, early mobilization also has disadvantages. The main reason for not starting my physiotherapy a day or two after surgery was that the scar that had formed would be larger, and consequently re-ruptures would be more common. Therefore, I was advised to rest during the first three to seven days to allow the scar tissue to gain strength. Subsequently, mobilization within pain-free limits was initiated. [49]

The first couple of days post-surgery saw me pretty much confined to bed. From day three, I was able to move around a little more in my wheelchair. In the beginning, I was able to wheel myself between my bed space and the toilet, thereafter progressing to the rest of the ward, down to Radiology and the hospital shop, albeit with the help of a ward assistant. However, my leg was still horizontally extended out from the wheelchair as I had to keep it slightly elevated lest it give me pain. This was due to the microvascular blood flow and the inability at this stage of my blood being able to return at the same rate of flow as it was pumping down to my foot. It was time to start rehabilitation.

---

[49] *"Muscle injuries: biology and treatment," American Journal of Sports Medicine, vol. 33, no. 5, pp. 745–764, 2005*

On the first day of my rehabilitation, I had arranged to start the session at 2:00pm, so just prior to that, I picked up the nurse-call handset and informed the duty nurse that it was time for my rehabilitation session. I then grabbed the ice pack on my bed, along with a half litre pet bottle of water and donned my slippers, before easing myself into my wheelchair. A ward assistant accompanied me to the rehabilitation centre and pushed me along the corridors, past the nurse station and up to the three large lifts. When a lift arrived, she wheeled me in and pressed the B1 button. When the lift doors opened, I was backed out and led out of the lift hall where we turned right and followed alongside the rehabilitation gym. There were large windows all the way along, which enabled me to see inside the gym and view everything going on there. As we continued alongside the gym, we ended up at the administration reception for rehabilitation. The assistant kindly informed the receptionist on the desk I was Mr. Smyth of the eighth floor and after some quick input on the screen in front of her, the receptionist handed me a large, plastic-embossed yellow card. As I was wheeled in through the entrance to the rehabilitation gym, we made a quick stop at an alcohol gel dispenser where I disinfected my hands.

As I rubbed the antibacterial lotion into my hands, I could clearly see to my right, a secluded area where several patients were completing a variety of neurological physiotherapy coordination exercises. Directly in front of me were seven or eight elderly patients parked in wheelchairs, quietly and uniformly waiting in turn to be attended to. A couple of them were wirelessly connected to an mobile ECG machine. When we moved off again, I could see four or five elderly persons to my left, lying or sitting up on long, wide padded benches and as we continued and turned ninety degrees to the right, a few more were lying on a series of pink benches. Moving past them, I was manoeuvred to the left and then immediately right, in front of a set of three benches, which formed a square. Here, I was introduced to my *"Rehabiri Sensei"*, my physiotherapist, and promptly handed her my yellow rehabilitation card.

Ms. Fujishima would be my physiotherapist for the duration of my rehabilitation. She immediately apologised in a slightly humorous fashion for her *"baby English"* to which I laughed and responded in Japanese that it was marvelous she could speak some English but that I could also speak in her language so communication wouldn't be an issue. Referring to her name badge, I asked if it was acceptable to call her by her first name but she asked me to refer to her as *"Fujishima Sensei"* or just *"Sensei"*, the latter meaning teacher or instructor. The ward assistant then left and I pulled myself up onto the bench, making sure the wheelchair brakes were on.

My physiotherapy, it was confirmed would be started gradually. I learned that *Isometric* training (type of strength training in which the joint angle and muscle length do not change during contraction) would be followed by *isotonic* training (form of muscle training where the muscle contracts and shortens, giving movement) and isotonic training by *isokinetic* training (exercise performed with a specialized apparatus that provides variable resistance to a movement, so that no matter how much effort is exerted, the movement takes place at a constant speed) once the respective exercises could be performed without pain.[50]

Fujishima Sensei got me to start off with some exercises to increase the range of motion in both my ankle and knee. With the aid of a special metal rehabilitation angle ruler, she first of all measured the maximum angle my leg would bend at the knee which, in my case, turned out to be seventy degrees. It seemed I needed to work towards being able to fully bend my leg back one hundred and eighty degrees. That would take some time but time was something I was more than willing to give to get my leg working again. For

---

[50] *"Muscle injuries: biology and treatment," American Journal of Sports Medicine, vol. 33, no. 5, pp. 745–764, 2005*

most of that first session, I did several sets of twenty leg bends, reaching the point of pain each time, with five minute rest intervals in-between.

During the rest periods, I was able to take in that area of the gym and what was happening around me. I could see to my left, in the centre of the room, a square, half-walled section which served as a place to obtain ice, water and towels. In front, slightly left and right of me were another forty benches, most of them occupied. This area of the gym was busy but different to that I had passed on the way in. The area I was in was full of younger people, mostly females, who had sustained sports-related injuries. As I learned later, most of those were ligament injuries to the knee and many of these patients were going through post knee surgery rehabilitation. This may not be surprising as Japanese students tend to focus a high percentage of their time and energy on sports activities. In fact, the growth of sport in Japan owes itself largely to colleges and sport has a close meaning to *"Do"* in Japan, meaning *"duty"* or *"the way"*[51], which is probably a major reason why Japan is such a strong contender in the Olympic games.

At the end of the session, Fujishima Sensei handed me a photocopy with several illustrations on it. These were the basic exercises I would follow for the duration of my rehabilitation. The first session lasted

---

[51] *http://www.humankinetics.com/acucustom/sitename/Documents/DocumentItem/6449.pdf*

just ninety minutes. I thanked her, adding that I looked forward to my next session the following day at the same time and then carefully levered myself into my collapsible wheelchair and headed back towards the Rehabilitation entrance, remembering to use the automatic antibacterial gel dispenser before heading back to the lift. This would be my daily routine every afternoon for the next two months.

My rehabilitation had barely begun when my cefazolin (prescribed antibiotic) cross-reaction kicked in, so consequently I was in no fit state to do rehabilitation during that period. In fact, I was essentially absent from rehabilitation for over a week. When I felt capable enough, I spent two days performing the exercises from the sheet Fujishima Sensei had provided for me while I was confined to bed. Given the importance of getting back to a proper rehabilitation regime, I was cleared to disconnect from the heparin infusion pump before heading down to rehabilitation each day. It was such a relief each time not to be connected to both that unit and the intravenous antibiotics.

On my return to rehabilitation, Fujishima Sensei was quite surprised to hear what had happened to me; during the interval. She was shocked to learn I had suffered a severe reaction to the antibiotics resulting in a rash all over my body together with a period of high fever and that I had been subjected to a biopsy. I told her about being intravenously attached twenty four hours a day to a heparin dosage control machine. She was also very concerned to learn that my CT scan had revealed three distinctive emboli resulting in the diagnosis of distal venal thrombosis. Nevertheless, she was happy that I had returned and could resume my physiotherapy sessions.

I started where I left off and continued with the knee raising exercises. With the angle measuring tool alongside my leg after three sets, I could clearly see that I had improved, which lifted my spirits. However, unsurprisingly, it took many hours of physiotherapy for my leg to be able to bend to its normal position. Bending my leg was the easy part. I needed to be able to bend my foot to its full range of motion, forward and backward and that was proving really difficult. I did a variety of other exercises each of which were designed to help me reach the normal range of motion in my ankle, so that when lying with my legs flat against the bench, I would be able to pull both feet up in line with each other. I was about four centimetres short of being able to do that with my injured leg although I could easily do so if I pulled my foot up with my hand. No matter how much I tried though, with just the muscles in my leg, that four centimetre gap seemed impossible to close and I could feel the sensation of strain in my shin leg muscles. Aside from suffering from muscle atrophy, it felt as though there was some kind of tight leather band preventing the muscles of my upper foot from moving up further, to close that four centimetre gap. At first, Fujishima Sensei thought it was likely to be one of the distal surgical locking screws that was holding my intramedullary rod in place, at the base of my tibia *where tibia meets tarsals*. This seemed to make sense as the area around the screw head incision point was inflexible. Dr. Tsuchiya thought this might also be the case and suggested if it was the muscle on either side of the screw head, they would soon work loose upon regular massage. This may have been part of the problem but it occurred to me that the real problem may have extended from that point to most of the way up my shin.

The problem was that when I moved my foot up, the muscles from my cruciate ligament up to my tibialis anterior did not feel flexible and independent from tissue and skin. Imagine a thick slice of beef with the subcutaneous tissue and skin still attached and how that skin moves freely up and down with the fingers. That was how my right leg was meant to feel, just as my uninjured left leg had. When I placed my fingers on the shin of my left leg and firmly moved up and down, the skin moved with my fingers, but when I tried with the right leg, there was resistance. It felt like trying to rub the skin on a raw potato. Similarly, as in my case, skin and muscle were firm and lacked flexibility. When I moved my right foot down as far as it would go without pain, I could feel the strain on my *extensor hallucis longus* (a long thin muscle situated on the shin that extends the big toe and dorsiflexes and supinates the foot) right up to my *tibialis anterior* (one of the thick fleshy anterior crural muscles of the leg, situated on the lateral side of the tibia). The area around my wound, where *superior extensor retinaculum* (the ligament that binds down the extensor tendons proximal to the ankle joint) meets *peroneus brevis* (the more superficial of the two lateral muscles of the leg) was not expanding and contracting as smoothly as it should. All the exercises I was doing were designed to strengthen these muscles and bring them back into operation.

For the first few weeks, I had been visiting the rehabilitation gym each day in the wheelchair that was assigned to me, initially with my right leg extended but a week after my intramedullary surgery, I was able to officially discard the 'L' shaped seat extension and ride with both legs down on the foot-rests. I had mastered manoeuvring and was able, without assistance, to progress from my bed to the hospital shop and cafe downstairs to start supplementing the predictable hospital food on offer. My daily morale booster was to bring a hot cup of tea up to my room after each rehabilitation session as there was a dire lack of hot water facilities in the ward. It was very convenient to get around in this manner and although I strengthened the muscles in my arms wheeling myself around, I was keen to get onto crutches.

The first day I was issued crutches, L size, by one of the nurses, just prior to a physiotherapy session, I propped them under my wheelchair, ready to take down to the rehabilitation gym. Near the end of the session on that day, Fujishima Sensei, my physiotherapist, adjusted them for me and I practiced walking around the gym with them after three o'clock, when the majority of people had finished their session. At first, I needed to bend my knee slightly to ensure my foot was not touching the floor. I would start off by doing a couple of rounds, then rest and elevate my leg against the large square pillar behind me to allow the flow of blood to return and reduce the swelling and redness. Although I could now move around like this with the assistance of crutches, moving between the rehabilitation gym and the ward was too risky and also exhausting for me, so I needed to use the wheelchair for a longer period of time until I became stronger and more confident with the crutches. Initially, it took a lot of practise to become accustomed to the feeling of placing just a quarter of my body weight on the leg. However, about a week or so later, I was able to do this and finally place the 25% load safely on my leg without risk of further injury.

It felt quite strange at first, placing my right foot down on the ground. It hadn't been on the ground since the time I stepped onto my bike and it felt so weak and useless. This was the first real hurdle for me though and as well as a marked physical progression, a revelation from being tied to a wheelchair, it was the clear beginning of learning to walk again. However, I needed to be really careful and control the weight load I was placing on my leg with every single step I made. Fujishima Sensei set up a measuring device to check that for me. There were several of these around the gym. Essentially, the device was an orange wooden platform approximately eight centimetres off the ground, about a metre wide and large enough to be able to stand on with both feet. On the one I used, there was a set of kilogram scales recessed into the frame so that the top of the scales was flush with the wooden surface. So each time around three o'clock, I would move over to this little stage and step onto it with my right leg placed on top of the scales. I would then shift my weight slightly to the right until the scales read twenty kilogrammes, which equated to 25% of my total body weight. The purpose here was to accurately determine what a specific percentage, i.e., 25% of my body weight, felt like on my injured leg. Anything over that specification would not be considered safe practice and could result in further injury until I received my physiotherapist's approval.

After a few times, I would practise without looking at the scales and then compare how close I was to my target. It was not easy at first, but eventually I felt confident that I knew what 25% felt like. Then I would move off the scales and walk reasonably slowly with the crutches until I made a full round, which would bring me back to the scales. The initial target was three sets of five rounds with a five minute rest interval. Each time I returned to the scales, I would go through the same procedure to check the weight load, making sure I wasn't placing more than a 25% kilogram force on the injured leg. The other important factor here was that I had a titanium rod running down the length of my tibia and aside from possibly falling over from any attempt to walk on anything in excess of 25% at that stage, due to muscle atrophy, I would probably not be able to feel any pain indication from significantly added weight. However, the obvious danger here was that my tibia, although shattered, was starting to repair itself and any excess force that could not be supported by my skeletal muscles could very easily damage the bone again and I wouldn't necessarily be able to feel that damage. The progression of load bearing on my leg was directly as a result of increasing strength and growth of bone callus, which was taken from the images on my weekly X-rays and confirmed by Dr. Tsuchiya.

Each Thursday afternoon, I would visit Radiology where lateral and anterior-posterior images of my leg would be taken. On Friday mornings or after the weekend, depending on priorities and workflow between the Radiology Department and the team that did the data processing, Dr. Tsuchiya would confirm the appropriate time to increase load bearing. Additionally, Fujishima Sensei was able to call up my X-ray images from a screen in her area of the gym. From the anterior-posterior images, there was no clear callus growth visibly extending the two millimetre gap fracture over my tibia but from the lateral images, callus growth was clearly appearing on the internal ends of the bone fragments, helping to create a union with the other sections of bone. Without signs of increasing callus growth on the ends of the bone, it would not be advisable to increase the weight loads.

Having become familiar with what a 25% load on my injured leg felt like, it was now time to leave my wheels in the room and commute to the gym on crutches, though I was advised by Fujishima Sensei to use the wheelchair if I was moving between floors to visit friends in other wards.

Progressing to 50% was again a remarkable achievement for me and all the closer to being able to walk properly, with crutches. Again, I would check the load bearing on the scales stage before each round, getting a sense for what fifty kilogramme force felt like on my injured leg. By this stage, my leg was not feeling as painful after each set in the vertical position. The inflammation was reducing and the time that it took for my leg to return to a somewhat normal colour after elevation was becoming shorter. Another milestone for my recovery was that I could finally say *sayonara* to my wheelchair. Thankfully, I was now left with a little more space around my bed.

One day, while still in the half weight-bearing stage, I noticed that my big toe had a slightly purple tinge to it and was becoming acutely sensitive to pain. I didn't think much of it until the following morning when it became more hyperalgesic and the purple colour had spread. It looked and felt like a bruise but instead of changing colour, as is the case in normal bruising, the purple colour continued to spread across my toe and was painful to touch. I couldn't recall any recent trauma to that area and after showing Dr. Tsuchiya, he wasn't sure what was causing it, other than it was possibly a side effect of the anticoagulant, warfarin. He arranged for an X-ray that afternoon and from the X-ray, he noticed that there was a tiny, non-recent fracture at the distal end of my first metatarsal. He thought this fracture may have been related to the bruising and suggested the condition would probably reduce and disappear in a few days. Within a week, it had disappeared but I was eager to know exactly what the problem was since I could only relate the fracture to a slight injury at the driving school earlier in February. So, with plentiful research, I conducted my own diagnosis and reached what I thought was an admirable conclusion. What I had suspected I had was a cholesterol embolism, commonly known as Purple Toe Syndrome. However, as I also learned in the course of my research, a cholesterol embolism is not a straightforward diagnosis as clinical documentation of the syndrome is not conclusive, although it does show correlation with warfarin. Further discussion with Dr. Tsuchiya confirmed my diagnosis when I saw him later as an out-patient.

What is known is that cholesterol embolism occurs when cholesterol is released, usually from an atherosclerotic plaque and travels along as an embolism within the bloodstream to other places in the body, where it obstructs blood vessels. Most commonly this causes skin symptoms, depending on the site at which the cholesterol crystals enter the bloodstream.

This phenomenon of embolisation of cholesterol was first recognized by the Danish pathologist, Dr. Peter Ludvig Panum and published in 1862.[52]

Embolism to the legs is known to cause purple discoloration of the toes, which was exactly what was happening to my big toe. These are small infarcts due to tissue necrosis which usually appear black, and areas of the skin that assume a somewhat marbled pattern known as ***livedo reticularis*** and is usually accompanied by severe pain.[53] Furthermore, it is known that cholesterol embolism can develop after administration of anticoagulant medication that decreases blood clotting. It is believed they probably lead to cholesterol emboli by removing blood clots that cover up a damaged atherosclerotic plaque; further leading to cholesterol-rich debris entering the bloodstream.[54] Clinical presentation of cholesterol embolization syndrome is often a combination of signs and symptoms specific to end-organ damage and a systemic inflammatory response. These crystals trigger an inflammatory response after they lodge in the small arteries of the target organ.[55]

---

52 *"Experimentelle Beitrage zur Lehre von der Embolie". Virchows Arch Pathol Anat Physiol (in German) 1862, 25 (5–6): 308–310*

53 *"Atheroembolic renal disease". J. Am. Soc. Nephrol. 12 (8): 1781–7*

54 *"Atheroembolic renal disease". J. Am. Soc. Nephrol. 12 (8): 1781–7. PMID*

55 *http://circ.ahajournals.org/content/122/6/631.full*

Findings on general investigations, such as blood tests, are not specific for cholesterol embolism, which makes diagnosis difficult. The main problem is the distinction between cholesterol embolism and *vasculitis* (inflammation of the small blood vessels), which may cause very similar symptoms, especially the skin discolouration.[56]

By mid August, I was able to progress from 50% loading to 75% loading, again getting up on to the scales to confirm the target percentage practised. It was only during my final week in rehabilitation that I was able to practise for the very first time in almost three months, walking without crutches. A glorious moment indeed. I walked as normally as I could past the people who were lying or sitting on the benches either side of me and I felt wonderfully free, but at the same time, I had been walking with the aid of my crutches for so long that it felt very strange without them. I did several circuits around the gym, not having to step onto the weight stage to check the load bearing, and then rested up. I learned to walk up the rehabilitation double-sided dummy staircase that had six 30cm steps with 10cm rises on one side and three 20cm steps with 15cm rises on the other, another small achievement.

However, after several sets, I started to feel pain in my knee and the area around the surgical screw

---

56 *"Atheroembolic renal disease". J. Am. Soc. Nephrol. 12 (8): 1781–7*

incision. There was a distinctively sensitive area in one particular spot right above the right proximal locking screw, but that only displayed sharp pain when depressed with my finger. The main problem was the increasing pain at the front of my knee, particularly vertically down my patellar tendon. One of the most common problems associated with tibial nailing, is chronic anterior knee pain.[57]

I began to walk with an uncontrollable limp again and normal strides were causing pain so I was forced to take shorter steps. My Physiotherapist, Fujishima Sensei thought it possibly related to the right lateral proximal surgical locking screw, since there was distinctive pain in a specific spot. When Dr. Tsuchiya briefly examined it in the early evening, he agreed that diagnosis could be the underlying cause of the pain but reserved judgement, believing there might be another reason and said he would examine me a few days later. Unfortunately, I didn't get to see him again as by that time I was discharged from hospital. Meanwhile, Fujishima Sensei asked me if I was able to tip toe on both feet, which I could do with ease, but when I tried to tip toe on just my right leg, I found it simply impossible. She thought that the knee pain was not so significant as it was not part of the trauma area, but gave me some new exercises to try which she thought

---

[57] *Reamed intramedullary nailing of the femur: 551 cases. J Trauma 1999;46:392–9*

would eventually help alleviate the problem. Essentially, they involved a ten minute session at a constant 30 watts (accurate measurement of energy output in the face of all resisting forces, to measure fitness) on one of the exercise bikes, followed by standing and simultaneously lifting both heels just two centimetres off the ground, fifty times. After a short rest period, I would walk over to the half wall in the centre of the room, next to the ice boxes and lean on top of the wall to absorb half of my body weight while I lifted my right heel off the ground just a centimetre or so. That I could do with the reduced weight. So fifty of those would constitute one of three sets.

Chapter Nine
Tai-in

When I finally returned home, I spent several hours researching the probable cause of my chronic anterior knee pain, sifting through many scholarly articles. What I discovered was that its incidence had been reported to be as high as 86%[58] and it came as no surprise to find that the site of the locking screw was mentioned as a primary cause as well as diffuse femoral pain from the presence of the intramedullary implant.[59] The most common causes of knee pain related to intramedullary nailing were the protrusion of distal locking screws and impingement of the nail on the patellar tendon and/or the articular surface of the tibial plateau.[60]

---

[58] *Anterior knee pain after intramedullary nailing of fractures of the tibial shaft: a prospective, randomized study comparing two different nail-insertion techniques. J Bone Joint Surg [Am] 2002;84-A:580–5*

[59] *Femoral shaft fractures treated by intramedullary nailing: a follow-up study focusing on problems related to the method. Injury 1995;26: 379–83*

[60] *Treatment of supracondylar femoral fractures with a retrograde intramedullary nail. Clin Orthop 1996;332:90–7*

However, although I could feel distinctive pain in the proximity of the locking screw when I pressed down on the area directly above the screw head, the pain I felt whilst walking came from the lower patellar tendon area, so I was interested to learn that the most frequent cause of pain in that specific area was in actual fact the longitudinal division of the patellar tendon during the *transtendinous* (through the tendon) approach per-surgery, the entry point of the nail and the protrusion of the nail proximally.[61] I also discovered the possibility that the proximal part of tibial nails can also provoke trauma to the patellar tendon and the fat pad.

Many authors of the research papers I read have suggested that both the *transtendinous* and *paratendinous* (around the tendon) approaches carry risks and are often related to post-operative knee pain. In the case of the transtendinous approach, the patellar tendon and the generously innervated retrotendinous fat pad are split longitudinally, as was the case in my surgery. In contrast, when the paratendinous approach is used, the patellar tendon, the fat pad and the gliding tissues are not divided but are repeatedly traumatised by retractors and reamers. Independent of the

---

[61] *Anterior knee pain after intramedullary nailing of fractures of the tibial shaft: a prospective, randomized study comparing two different nail-insertion techniques. J Bone Joint Surg [Am] 2002;84-A:580–5*

approach used, injury to the tendon and soft tissues is unavoidable and it is therefore believed that the degree of this per-operative trauma is the most important causative factor.[62]

Anterior knee pain has also been attributed to weakness of the thigh muscles. Neuromuscular inhibition of quadriceps and *gastrocnemius* (the large muscle on the back of the lower leg, that connects with the Achilles tendon and extends the foot) occurs after knee injury, lower-limb trauma, extensor mechanism injury and reduced weight-bearing.[63] However, researchers at St. James University Hospital in Leeds, England and The Royal Infirmary of Edinburgh, Scotland[64] believe that weakness of thigh muscles is actually the result and not the cause of anterior knee pain, as others have suggested.[65] Vaisto et al[66] observed that anterior knee pain after intramedullary nailing of fractures of the tibia may be related to deficiencies in

---

[62] *Anterior knee pain after intramedullary tibial nailing. Changgeng Yi Xue Za Zhi 1999;22:604–8*

[63] *Long-term quadriceps femoris functional deficits following intramedullary nailing of isolated tibial fractures. Int Orthop 2001;24:342–6*

[64] *http://www.bjj.boneandjoint.org.uk/content/88-B/5/576.short#ref-12*

[65] *Antergrade versus retrograde reamed nailing: a prospective randomized trial. Procs Annual Meeting of Orthopaedic Trauma Association Canada 1998*

[66] *Anterior knee pain and thigh muscle strength after intramedullary nailing of tibial shaft fractures: a report of 40 consecutive cases. J Orthop Trauma 2004;18:18–23*

the strength of the knee flexors.[67] No matter the cause, I would have to deal with this discomfort when I discharged from hospital.

During my final week in Kanto Rosai, I realised that not only had I been in the hospital for almost three months but that I had actually become use to it and the idea of being released into the real world was a big step. There was a lot to think about. My day-release a couple of weeks earlier served as a solemn reminder that things would not be as easy on the outside as they were in hospital. In contrast, the hospital environment was relatively safe. For one thing, there were only doctors, nurses, nursing staff, patients and visitors here and the pace of daily life was comfortable and relatively slow. Patients moved around in wheelchairs, on crutches, with walking frames, with walking sticks or just walked slowly. There was little chance of literally bumping into another person, patient or staff, except perhaps in the lift. There was no work to rush off to here, no train to catch and no clients to visit nor an expanding inbox filling with tiresome email correspondence. There were no social events or friendly gatherings to attend. We all just went about at our own pace, yet this slow pace and the environment just seemed so normal after a while.

---

[67] *Anterior knee pain and thigh muscle strength after intramedullary nailing of tibial shaft fractures: a report of 40 consecutive cases. J Orthop Trauma 2004;18:18–23*

This was, after all, the perfect environment for a wheelchair, crutches or a walking frame. The floor was flat, the corridors spacious and there were no obstacles to negotiate, except perhaps for the odd bed or parked-up nurse PC trolley. There were no tricky stairs to negotiate or unsecured cables to step over and the lifts were large enough to accommodate several patients in wheelchairs at a time. Help was always close by. There was no need to vacuum or brush the floor and no need to dust the surfaces, clean the windows, change the curtains or even turn the lights off at night. It was not necessary to change the bed linen nor hang it out to dry. There was no need to go shopping for food because there was no need to cook, which in turn meant there were no dishes to wash, therefore nothing to dry. The room temperature was comfortable. It never became too cold or even too hot and the relative humidity was always low and comfortable.

There was plenty of leisure time to be enjoyed, watching TV dramas and movies. I could spend time reading or patiently spend hours sketching and planning what I'd do when I left hospital. I had so much time to chat with other people and learn new things, laugh and share thoughts and opinions. I didn't have to work, which meant I didn't have to wait in line to catch an early morning train to be squashed onboard like a sardine and because I didn't have to play sardines, I didn't need to travel around the city from client to client, wearing out the soles of my good quality shoes. Most of all I had escaped the searing heat and its dripping humidity. Life had become easy and by default this easy life was saving me from spending, for not working meant I wasn't spending lots of money in Starbucks, in Tulleys, and in the fashionable world of Japanese department stores like Takashimaya. I didn't need to spend my hard earned cash in my favourite home centres or restaurants, craft shops or in electronic stores, seeking out the latest technologies. So I discovered for the short term, there were actually benefits to be had as an in-patient.

Most benefits don't last of course and it was time to give up this slow pace of life doing practically whatever I wanted to do to occupy myself. The time to trade that period of freedom in for a normal life was fast approaching and I had to prepare for the transition.

Of course, being released from hospital to return to the normality of life before trauma is undoubtedly exciting and something to really look forward to. Three months in hospital had stolen a part of my life, dusted the things I owned and placed them on the shelf for my return. It had grabbed my daily life and twisted this chunk of time into an unrecognisable shape, one that I was obliged to follow with a set of rules to which I was expected to adhere.

Although I had adequate insurance cover for the duration of my hospitalisation and recovery, I was nevertheless keen to return to work and normality. Being away from the work environment for three months was bound to have had an adverse effect on my clients' business arrangements as well as my employers and this was of great concern to me as at the point of discharge from hospital I had no idea when I would be likely to return to my business responsibilities. Being away from the work environment meant I was faced with a language that had gone rusty on me and as a consequence, I struggled at times to adequately express and articulate myself.

I had to respect others whenever I created any kind of noise, especially at night. I had to spare generous consideration toward my neighbours when I turned on a light at night, when I coughed or sneezed or talked with my visitors and friends whilst at the same time, having to endure those very same things from others. I had to put up with the constant noise of nurses rushing around or attending to me, doctor visits, pharmacist visits, administration staff visits, ward assistant visits and other patients communicating with each other. I had to endure the incessant throat clearing episodes of old men, the blatant rumbling release of wind, the excessive coughing episodes and the dreadful sleep-depriving snoring duets straining like trombones and trumpets out of sync with each other. I had to endure sleeping in a narrow bed that was barely long enough for me on a mattress that was as soft as a picnic blanket in that peace park across the road. I had to make do with the small space around my bed and the desperate lack of storage space for my clothes and other necessities, and I had to share a toilet with several other people who didn't particularly leave it as clean as I had left it for them.

I needed a haircut but couldn't visit my hairdresser of six years. I missed being able to nip down to the convenience store and although I saved around a thousand dollars in hot earl grey teas and cappuccino coffees, I really missed Starbucks. I missed just driving through the city in the car, jogging along the raised grass banks of the Tamagawa River or just walking across the splendour of Marukobashi bridge. I missed watching the sun setting behind the tall reed grasses along the banks of the gently flowing river and the beautiful moon as it glowed above the commandeering skyline of majestic Musashikosugi. Whether in the midst of morning, in the heart of afternoon or in the quiet of night when the lights were switched off, I always had to don my earphones when I wanted to watch those TV dramas and movies and for the most part, it was not possible to enjoy a relaxing cup of tea or coffee as there was no hot water nearby. The almost intolerable limits of food choice and freedom were starting to nibble around the edges of my tolerance. It was time to step back into the real world. Most of all I longed for the comforts of my own home, the laughter of my beautiful daughter, Lilian and sharing family life with my wife, Noriko.

I had gone through what I hope will be only a once in a lifetime experience but it wasn't a totally unpleasant experience. Rather it was an experience that started with pain and ended with relieve but amidst that black and white of my in-patient months I had inadvertently embarked on a journey, an experience and a time in a different world. It was a world I didn't really belong to yet I settled in well and I came to understand and respect this world.

Epilogue

As I sit at home now, putting the finishing touches to *"From Sertão to Surgery"* in the final weeks of December, 2014, after having collected my dignity at the hospital gates, I can reflect upon my unplanned quarter of a year's stay in hospital from outside the walls, deep in the heart of the real world, a world that seems so far from where I was only a matter of weeks ago. Each day, my story feels more like a fading tale than a journey that is etched on my memory, but the pain and trauma of my fractured leg, the anxiety and discomfort of the edematous suffering I endured throughout my period of *'allergia cephalosporium'* and the worrying, tiring time I had in dealing with blood clots I shall of course never forget.

In the course of my experience over the months since my accident, I have discovered a great many things about my body, of the medicines I was administered, and of myself since that fateful day in June when my BMW g650 GS Sertão decided to fall on me with the equivalent weight of 74 red house bricks. I unintentionally embarked upon a remarkable journey and in so doing, I hope to have shared with you some sense of what it's like as a Westerner, to stay in a Japanese hospital over a lengthy period of time. Throughout this account, I have endeavoured to share a knowledge of the clinical practices I endured as an orthopaedic trauma patient, while simultaneously bringing into the story a very small slice of the complicated world of medicine.

I discovered the important role physiotherapy plays in muscle recovery and the reality of just how long it really takes to recover from a fractured tibial injury. I found myself among a unique group of people in the area of the rehabilitation gym I was in, unique in the sense that we all had something in common; we had all been subjected to some kind of accident and we had all at some point suffered pain. All of us needed to go through some combination of those isotonic, isometric and isokinetic exercises and we all walked around the gym as we increased our strength once again, ready to be signed-off for our re-entry into the real world.

As of December 2014, my knee still gives me some pain when I walk and as an alternative to performing another small surgery to remove or re-adjust the proximal locking screws, Dr. Tsuchiya has prescribed me, a three months supply of acetaminophen, an analgesic-antipyretic from the paracetamol family of pain killers in order to reduce the pain of full knee rehabilitation. However, to reduce my dependency on the acetaminophen, I have decided to use a walking stick for the next few months. Having analysed the evidence of bone regeneration shown on the lateral X-ray images and the fact that there is still a gap between the bone fragments shown on the A.P. X-ray image, I have theorised the cause of my anterior knee pain is a consequence of the contraction of the anterior side of my leg at the trauma site as it is compressed with each stride of full body weight, which in turn is pulling my patellar tendon across the heads of the surgical screws which lock the top of the intramedullary rod in place. I believe the use of the walking stick will help reduce the full weight on my right leg and allow the bone to regenerate without the further complication of added pressure and movement. I will suggest my theory to Dr. Tsuchiya when I see him for my next consultation.

I can only hope that this will be the final solution and the 'final chapter' of my pain, though it will not be the 'final chapter' of my leg trauma. A year from now, I may agree to having the surgical locking screws removed and in three years time, when my tibia has completely returned to its pre-Sertão state, I may choose to check-in to hospital 'paradise' again for another week or two to have the intramedullary rod removed. Having to go through rehabilitation again is a daunting thought but for the time being, I am looking forward to once again hiking in the mountains of Japan.

Hiking has been a great past-time of mine since I was a teenager. At school, I would enjoy short educational trips into the countryside to better understand the history of my country through the many historical sites and artifacts that are the remnants of British history. When I was just thirteen years old, I remember once staying in the old mining town of Allendale, deep in the Northumbrian countryside, where we hiked across the boggy wetness to visit what was left of the slate stone smelter houses and the ruined sandstone chimneys that once towered above them. It was in these smelter houses that thousands of tons of lead ore were once smelted down into lead and it was here that we'd be able to find plentiful lead ore samples. Walking across this terrain for miles to visit these places, left our boots soaking wet and our waterproof trousers splattered with the mud from the hoard of dirt track puddles we had to negotiate, but I loved it. This was my first real taste of adventure and unbeknown to me at the time, the very beginning of a long life of hiking and adventure that would continue to inspire me throughout my life.

I recall the time a few years later while still in my teens when I planned a hiking and camping trip across the magnificent Northumberland countryside. My cousin and I packed a tent, sleeping bags, roll mats, waterproof clothing and cooking utensils in our large framed rucksacks and with a map, set out to walk from the old Roman Wall in the western side of Newcastle upon Tyne, through the old Roman town of Morpeth and all the way up through Rothbury towards Berwick-upon-Tweed. Both of us learned a lot from that trip, not least the importance of having adequate rain gear and footwear.

I pursued my passion for hiking adventures throughout my teenage years and into my twenties, adventure that took me across the Cairngorm mountain range in Northern Scotland, the Cuillins on the Isle of Skye, across the hills of the Outer Hebrides, the winter white topped mountains of Glen Affric and to the summit of Scotland's second highest mountain, *An Teallach,* in Wester Ross. My experience in hiking and adventure served me well through my Army training, its strength and confidence helping me achieve the honour of holding the Queen's Commission after passing out from the Royal Military Academy Sandhurst and being commissioned as a Second Lieutenant (infantry) into the 3rd Battalion Highlanders.

Not long after settling in to my new life here in Japan, I sought out adventure which I found in an outdoor club called the International Adventure Club (IAC). During its peak membership of some 450 members, I served two consecutive years as President and another three years as Adventure Coordinator. Twenty years later, I am still an active member of the club, having enjoyed many years of hiking, camping and other adventures.

With all this adventure experience, and having owned a Yamaha DT125 LC trail bike when I was living in Scotland, perhaps it will come as no surprise that I pursued my adventurous desire to ride the ultimate in *'enduro'* motorcycles when the chance arose. I have no regrets towards my having pursued motorcycle lessons in the U.K. and in Japan or indeed of losing balance of such a beautiful but heavy machine, one which caused me to spend three precious months of my life in hospital, stealing many months, and possibly years, from my passion for hiking and the outdoors.

Many of the friends who came to visit me in hospital were surprised to discover that I never once felt depressed at my situation. During my entire stay in hospital I found the determination and mental strength to fight against the physical pain and trauma to which my body was being subjected. Whenever I experienced discomfort, allergic reaction or bad news, I would just dig my heels in deeper and stand my ground, with a committed smile upon my face, for as Aristotle once remarked, "*The ideal man bears the accidents of life with dignity and grace, making the best of circumstances.*"[68]

As for my Sertão, it has once again inflicted pain upon me, this time not a physical one but a mental pain for as sad and as difficult as it is, I promised my wife, Noriko, (*somewhat under duress*), that I would sell my beautiful BMW g650 GS Sertão and give up my BMW biking dream and that I did, right back to the source. My bike once again sits in the showroom window of BMW Motorrad Haneda on Kanpachi Dori, waiting for some lucky new owner to discover this unique adventure on two wheels.

[68] *http://www.brainyquote.com/quotes/quotes/a/aristotle130621.html*

Acknowledgements

I should like to thank Orthopaedic Surgeons, Dr. Tsuchiya, Dr. Hyodo and Dr. Okazaki; the Dermatologist, Dr. Kitajima; nurses of A Teams 8F East and 5F West Nurse Stations and my Physiotherapist, Fujishima Sensei, of Kanto Rosai Hospital, Musashikosugi, Japan for the support and patient care that was afforded me during my period of hospitalisation. I should also like to thank my wonderful mother, Marie, who spent hours of her time via her MacBook Air editing my drafts whilst burning the midnight oil some 9,328 km away in the U.K. Mum provided constant support, knowledge and encouragement on a daily basis via her iPhone during my hospital stay and throughout my recovery period and kept me thinking positively, especially during my darkest moments. I also thank my long-suffering wife, Noriko and my beautiful daughter, Lilian for their constant visits and attention and for putting up with seeing me with my nose in my MacBook Air writing this book in the months following my discharge from hospital. My grateful thanks goes to the manager and other kind neighbours of the apartment complexes adjacent to my house, who came to my rescue on the morning of June 5th, 2014, helped me to safety and stayed with me while I waited the arrival of the ambulance. Finally, I thank my colleagues and all my good and loyal friends from the Tokyo 'International Adventure Club' who took time to travel to Musashikosugi to visit me in hospital, cheer me up and boost my morale.

Appendices

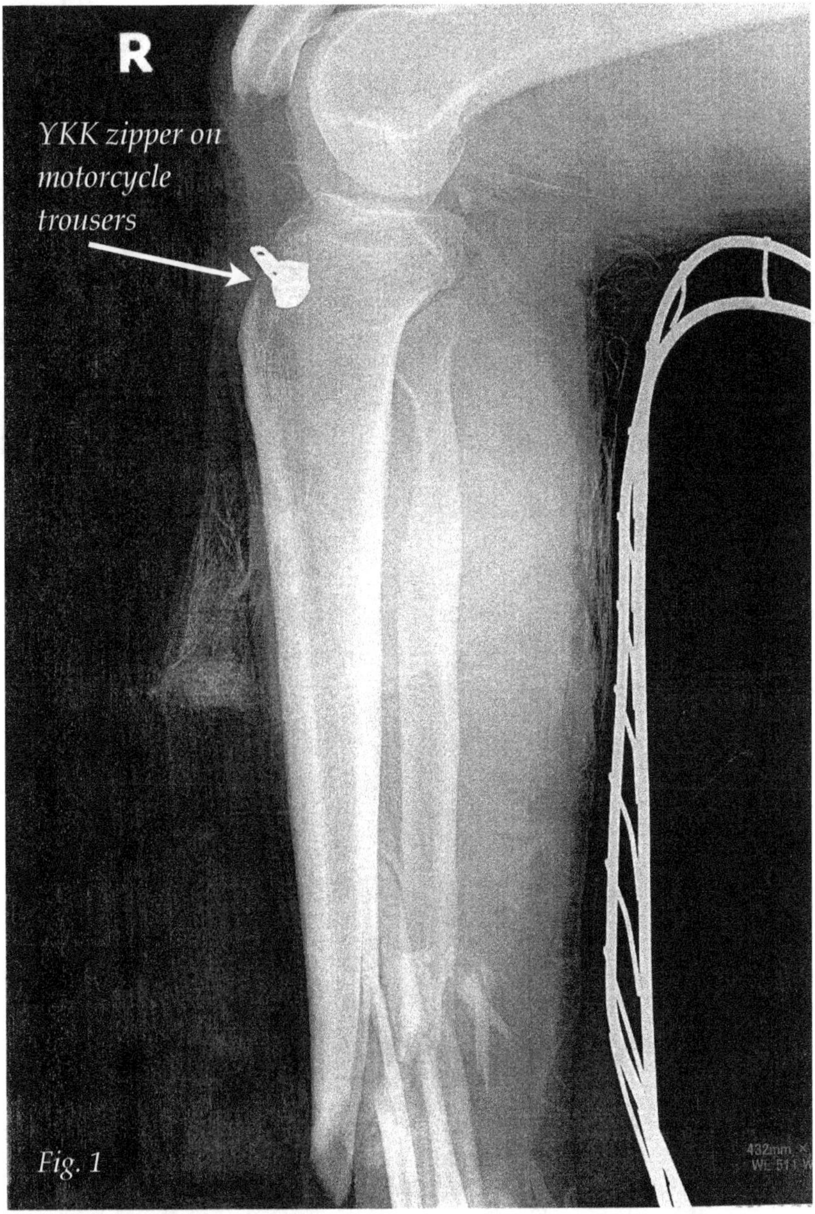

Lateral X-ray image (fig. 1) taken about one hour after arrival in E.R. The image shows the metal support used in the ambulance.

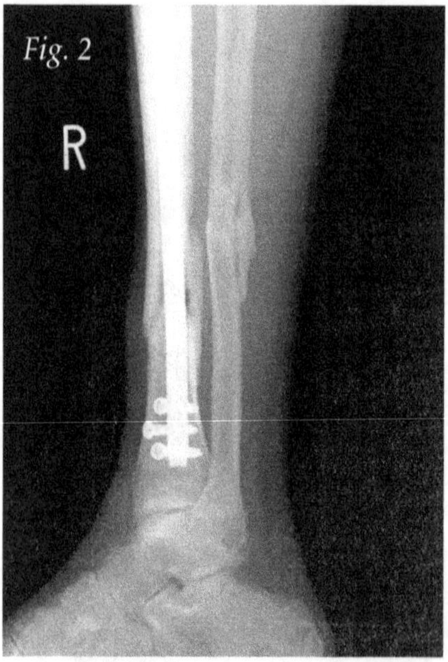

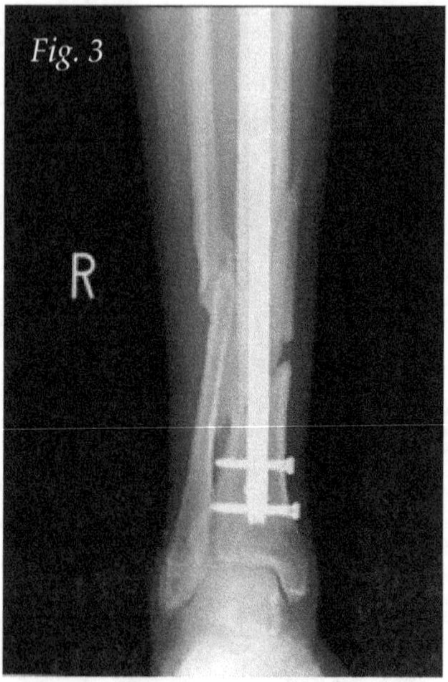

Lateral (fig. 2, left) and Anterior-Posterior (fig. 3, right) X-ray images taken on 16th October, 2014 and clearly showing the titanium intramedullary rod and surgical locking screws. The lateral image shows bone callus growth, fusing the tibia together. The Anterior-Posterior image on the right shows callus growth still needs to extend across the bone fragments. The X-ray image below (fig. 4) was taken on 31st July, 2014.

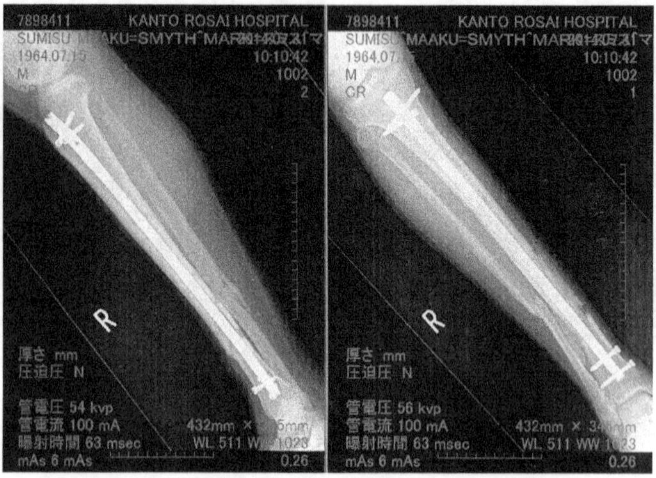

Fig. 4

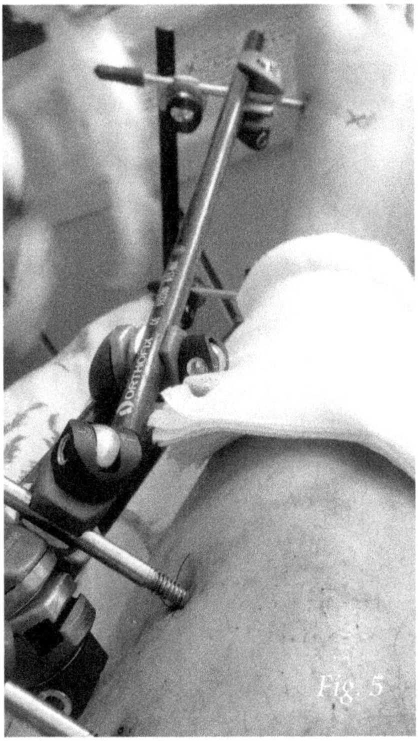

Fig. 5

The external fixation apparatus attached per-surgery on June 5th, 2014 to hold my tibia in place and stabilise the leg. The pins were screwed directly into the stable sections of bone to a depth of up to 8cm.

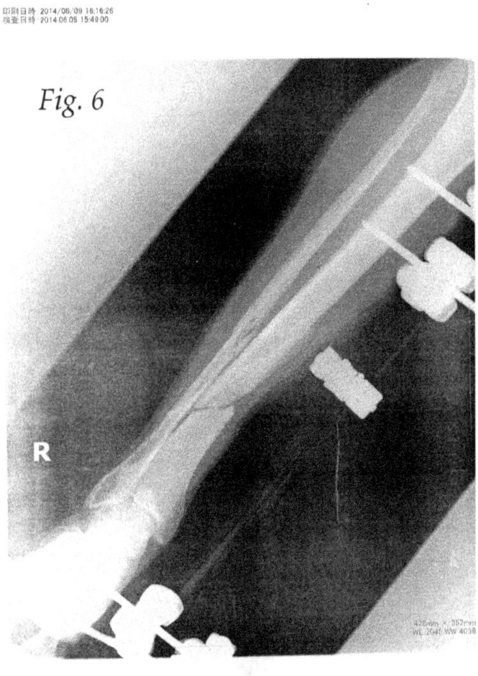

Fig. 6

Anterior-Posterior X-ray image taken after emergency operation, showing comminuted fracture stabilised with the external fixation apparatus.

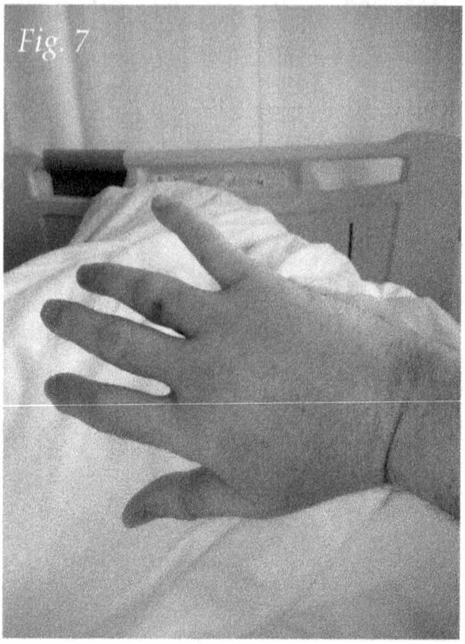

Fig. 7

The effects of my allergic reaction to Cefazolin antibiotic

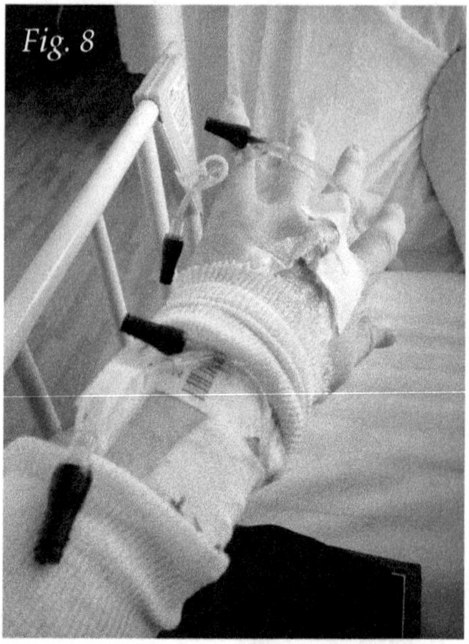

Fig. 8

My arm intravenously connected to heparin anti-coagulant and Daptamycin antibiotic.

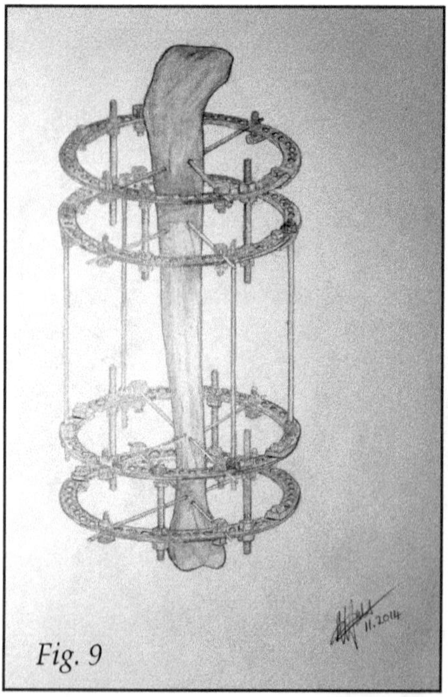

Fig. 9

The Ilizarov Apparatus

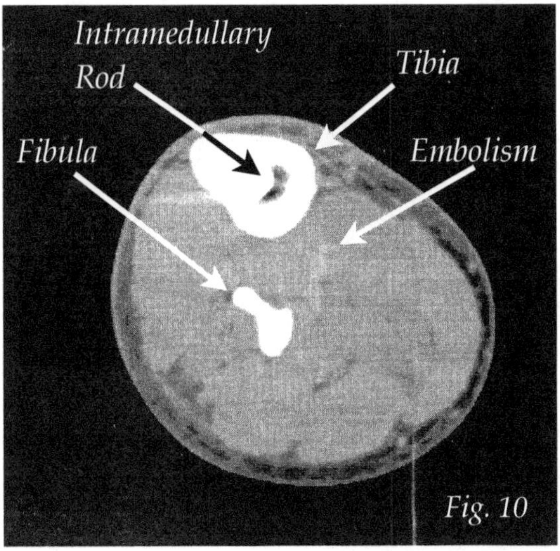

Fig. 10

A CT tamogram (fig.10) taken during the CT scan showing and looking up towards the top of the tibial shaft. An embolism can be seen near the top of the tibia. The white area in the middle of the tibia is the titanium rod.

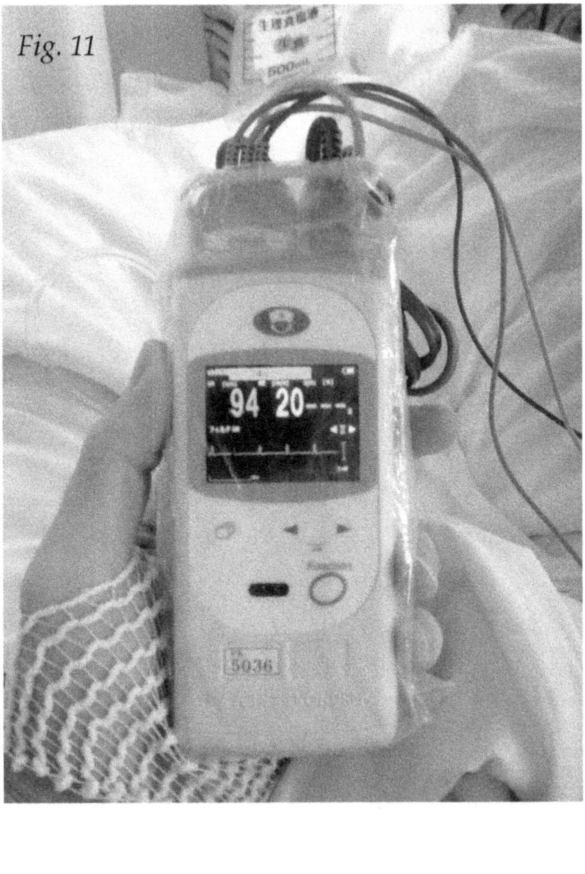

Fig. 11

Portable WiFi-enabled ECG device to which I was attached for two weeks.

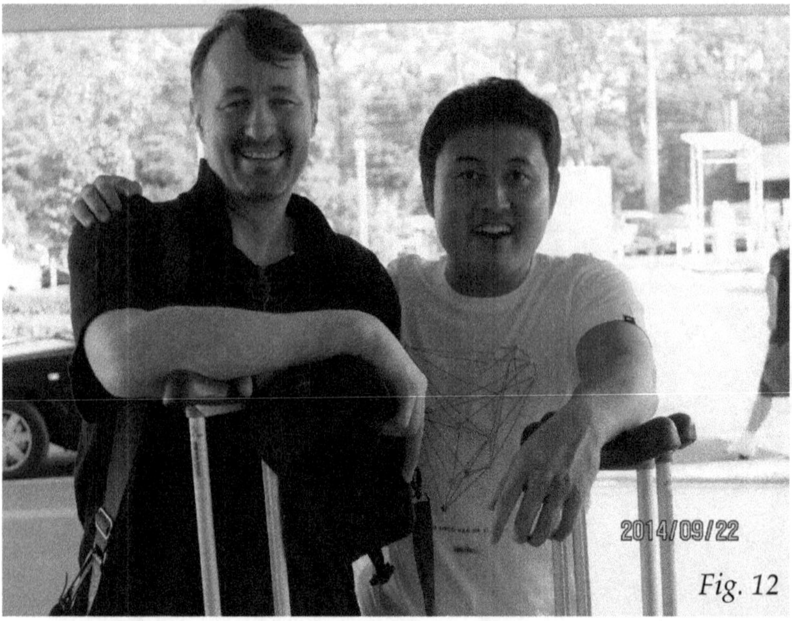

Fig. 12

New friends made whilst an in-patient at Kanto Rosai. Above (fig.12), the author (left) with Takeo Kubota. Below (fig.13), with Tora Andy, outside the Doutor Cafe we frequented daily.

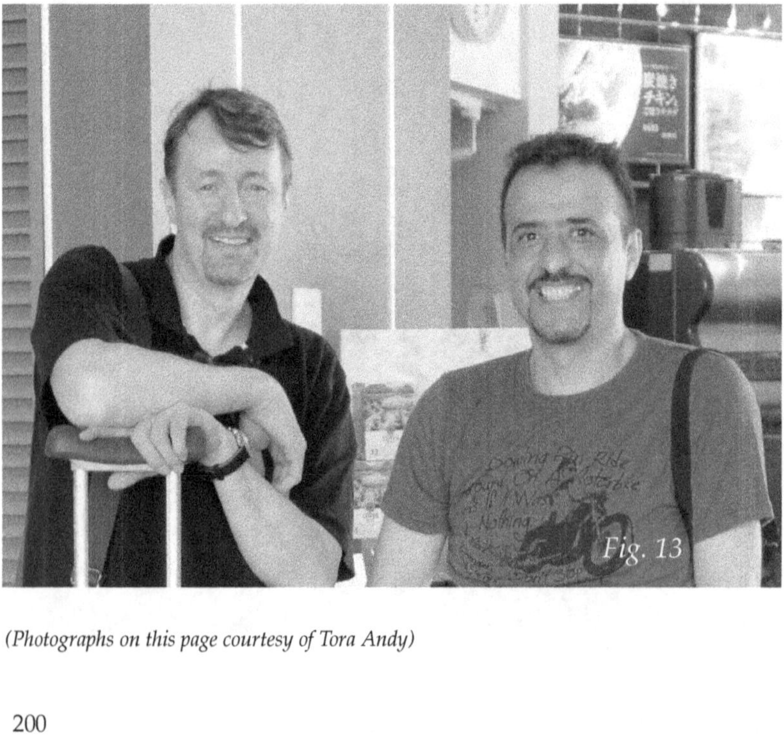

Fig. 13

(Photographs on this page courtesy of Tora Andy)

List of 47 Pharmaceutical Drugs Administered whilst at Kanto Rosai Hospital

Allegra® 60mg (fexofenadine)
Allelock® OD (olopatadine hydrochloride)
Amlodipine
Antebate® Ointment (Betamethasone Butyrate Propionate)
Atarax® P (Hydroxyzine embonate)
Atropne Sulphate 0.05%
Bridion® (sugammadex)
Brotizolam
Calonal® (Paracetamol)
Clindamycin
Cubicin® (Daptomycin)
Diprivan® (Propofol)
Durotep® (Fentanyl)
Ephedrine
Elieten® (Metoclopramide)
Epinephrine
Eslax® (Rocuronium Bromide)
Gaster® (Famotodine)
Gentacin® (Gentamicin sulfate)
Ibuprofen
Lincomycin
Locoid® (Hydrocortisone Butyrate)
Loxoprofen Sodium
Neomallermin TR (Chlorphenamine Maleate)
Novo Heparin (Heparin Sodium)
Olopatadine Hydrochloride
Oypalomin® (Iopamidol)
Pentagin (Pentazocine)
Povidone-iodine
Rebamipide
Xylocaine® (Lidocaine)
Rasenazolin® (Cefazolin Sodium)
Rinderon®-V (Betamethasone Valerate)
Ringer's Solution, Bicarbonated
Ropion® (Flurbiprofen axetil)
Saline
Sevofrane® (Sevoflurane)
Soldem3A
Solulact (Lactated Ringer's Solution)
Sulyugen F
Ultiva® (remifentanil Hydrochloride)
Vancomycin MEEK
Vidarabine
Voluven® (Hydroxyethyl Starch)
Warfarin
Xarelto®
Zolpidem Tartrate

www.ingramcontent.com/pod-product-compliance
Lightning Source LLC
Chambersburg PA
CBHW071424170526
45165CB00001B/388